If you think you are beaten, you are;
If you think you dare not you don't
If you like to win, but you think you can't
It is almost certain think you won't;

If you think you'll lose you've lost,
For out of the world we find
Success begins with a fellow's will-
It's all in the state of mind.

If you think you are outclassed, you are.
You've got to think high to rise.
You've got to be sure of yourself before
You can ever win a prize.

Life's battles don't always go
To the stronger or faster man;
But soon or late the man who wins
Is the man who thinks he can.

THE BOY WHO WANTED THE SKY

ARVIND AGGARWAL

ISBN: 9798865565468

CONTENTS

To *Meena,*

My Life

To *Shilpi & Vikash*

Our Light

To *Zara,*

Our All.

To *Meena,*

My Life

To *Shilpi & Vikash*

Our Light

To *Zara,*

Our All.

Foreword

From the agricultural heartland of Punjab, springs to life a fascinating tale - the life story of a young boy with boundless ambition that is matched with an extraordinary vision. As the reader turns over the pages of *The Boy who Wanted the Sky*, the central protagonist grows up to reveal a stubbornness of purpose and innovation of thought, blended in fair measure with intestinal fortitude; but most of all, an abiding love for family, friends and not least, humanity.

As we experience his challenges, his triumphs and failures; we revel in the courage, the fortitude and the humility with which each is met. Here is a refreshing story of a character who's real, versatile and will unapologetically try alternative paths where necessary; managing to carve success stories out of stumbling stones as he progresses towards his *raison d'etre* or *ikigai* - bringing home the elixir of quality healthcare to us all.

The author sees Healthcare as an important human right, much more than a service where access and quality of the care received is determined through the strength of wallet or influence.

India and many other countries with emerging economies have very large indigent populations. For governments - providing healthcare to large masses of populations - often poses an enormous challenge for a variety of reasons. Yet, it is not only the poorer countries that are seen to grapple with this problem, even in the wealthy United States of America - substantial portions of the population suffer severely restricted access to adequate healthcare.

And heartbreakingly, what we witnessed back in the 1990s when Dr. Aggarwal first introduced his Project, still continues to be true. But given the the technology boom today; Healthcare, or at least, the delivery of Healthcare need not be found lacking any longer. Consider the rural populations of India, Pakistan and Bangladesh - they are largely similar with respect to their limited or complete absence of accessibility to healthcare. It will be safe to say that if their general health remains low, there will be no way to lift them out of their poverty. Individuals as you, me and indeed, everyone of us needs to feel well enough. At all times.

And Dr. Arvind Aggarwal has designed a system that can self-implement delivery of healthcare - to serve the people, especially those ailing at the margins. A System that will effectively cut down the 'wait time'. Really trim down the travel and investigation time - so that the fatalities will gradually reduce until they die out entirely. Thereby heralding a Socialisation of Medicine.

In the pages of this book, the Doctor has revealed the blueprint of his mission to design and deliver the system to uplift the people. Through a self-sustaining mechanism. A system that will help raise the people's energy, their vitality so they can feel *well enough*. And truly empowered. Because so long as we feel well, we will work towards building our autonomy, ourselves.

The Doctor is determined to effect this long-awaited change - affordable and quality healthcare for all, instantly. And I hope we can join forces. Once you have read this book, I hope you have a serious think about how you might be able to help or support this noble endeavour.

- Bob Phillips

Part I

A Star is Born

Chapter 1

IN THE BATTLEFIELDS

Boom boom! Boom boom! Boom!!
Boommm!
Boom Boom!!

The deafening explosions had lasted well into the night. Air strikes became increasingly common during the Indo-Pak War of 1965. Lights couldn't be switched on after dark and schools and colleges remained closed for most of the year.

We were asked to carefully stick black carbon paper on all window panes so that the light does not escape.

Ambala Cantonment, where I was born on 8th June 1952, is one of the biggest cantonments in India that is geographically located very close to Pakistan (situated 200 km south of Lahore border and about exactly the same distance down from Delhi). Every evening, the siren sounded, asking people to 'black-out' and move to the trenches; warning, that there may be an air-raid, anytime, once the army detected planes crossing into India through radars.

The elders in the family would immediately switch off the lights around the house. My father explained that black-outs were conducted to prevent the enemy aircrafts from identifying their targets. He showed me how the headlights of our vehicles were horizontally half-painted in black, so their light beams deflected downwards to the ground.

Next morning, we would go to the sites to find the bombshells, that were dropped through the night and 'examine' the ravages of buildings that were now turned into ruins. I often saw railway racks, carrying heavy military equipment including heavy trucks and tanks passing by Ambala station. While we didn't realise it then, we were living in war zone. And every new day was a gift.

To prevent us from stealing outside to play, the elders would graphically relate how planes from Lahore came to Ambala, drop a bomb and go back, all within minutes.

The air was thick with 'the stories' of toys found on park benches that were actually bombs waiting to explode, Pakistani spies who were present amidst the crowds - in the marketplaces, in the hallways and in the lanes.

One day, a church, quite close to our house, was bombarded. It was an old church, adjoining the Pilots'

Mess, the Military Hospital and the Army Club. The air strike was intended at bombing the Pilots' Mess, but it had missed its target, ending up bombing the Church instead.

The blazing sight of giant red flames, escaping out of the tall minarets, before falling to the ground, and lighting up the expanse of the area cast a hypnotic spell upon my 13-year old eyes as I peered through the little corner of the window where the carbon paper had pealed.

Sometimes the planes would fly so low that you might want to duck your head lest you actually touch them. But there was no escaping the ominous whirring sound of the rotating wings.

My eldest brother was in Air Force and was posted in Ambala. He and some of his friends-colleagues shifted from the Pilots' Hostel to stay with us at this time.

In the massive open courtyard of our house, we dug out a Z-shaped trench, something of a hideout where we could seek refuge against bombardment. One of those days, when there was an air strike, we wanted to get into the trench. But we were in for a rude shock. Just as we entered, a pair of eyes gleamed in the dark, the body throbbing aggressively and looking to rip us apart. We froze with fear. I could feel a sudden emptiness in the pit of my stomach. She let out a belligerent stream of threatening guttural sounds that knocked the wind out of our lungs. And then, a fearsome growl followed that revealed two white rows of sharp canines looking for blood.

A particularly angry female dog who'd given birth to a litter of puppies in the dark trench and made it her home, saw us as the enemy.

And each time, we rushed into the trench for shelter against hostile air raids, she'd launch an attack on us.

Until she began to trust us.

* * *

At Poondri

One day, the army went around announcing for all civilians to vacate the town immediately, in view of the mounting security concerns.

We decided to go to Poondri, a village about 100 km from Ambala to live with a distant cousin of my father's, *Bade Tauji* (father's elder brother) *Tauji* ran a grocery store in the village but every morning, he would go to the fields to cut hay to feed the animals.

Tauji was a sturdy man with a moustache that seemed to twirl upwards on either side, filling out the empty space of his tanned cheeks. He was fond of the children and I used to love going with him into the fields to watch him use the massive cutter to cut hay. Just moving the cutter took a lot of strength. Whenever he sat down to rest awhile, it would be 'my turn' to clumsily brandish it about - my young heart utterly delighted at the prospect of growing great bicep muscles like *Tauji*.

* * *

Home

I was the ninth child to my parents who had an equal number of sons and daughters (five each).

At 6 am every morning, my mother would ready the

angeethee(earthen heater)and make tea. We were a big family. Anybody going into the kitchen would always return with two steaming cups or glasses of tea, the second was for anybody who he may barge into on the way . . .

The standard breakfast was always *parathas* (hand made Indian bread) and *aloo sabzi*(potato curry) followed by some more tea.

But of course, I would always want instead a *halwa* (semolina confectionary) or *chilla* (Indian pancake made of lentils) or *aalo poori* (potato curry and deep fried flour bread).

Grandfather had a *Kohlu* (an oil mill that manufactures oil from mustard seeds). Every morning, my father, father's elder brother and my grandfather went to the mill on their special vintage carriage'Victoria', drawn by a beautiful white steed greatly loved by the family.

Before he left home every morning, my father would give my mother money for household expenses. Those days, there were no currency notes. I would watch as he plunged his arm into a *potli* (cloth bag fastened with strings) and bring out, like a magician from his treasure bag, a fistful of jiggly shiny coins, placing them carefully into mother's palms . . . and no, counting was not customary.

My earliest recollection of all of us together is that of my father, uncle and grandfather returning from the oil mill; bringing home the day's earnings in shiny tin canisters. This would be emptied out on the carpet in the big drawing room for the children to count.

All of us children, with a solemn sense of purpose, would make separate heaps of one *Anna*, two *Anna's*, four *Anna's* (*Chawanni*), eight *Anna's* (*Athanee*) and a rupee (*Chandi ka rupiah*).

And most often, most of us would fall asleep while counting, with Mother putting us to bed.

Chapter 2

INVENTOR AT 13!

Summers in Ambala are utterly punishing.

My school summer vacation made this amply clear. The May heat is sweltering with a hot wind called 'Loo' blowing in our part of the world, often resulting in serious fatalities for those out in the sun. So, by afternoons, the streets wear a deserted look in an otherwise bustling city. I was in the 8th standard at school in 1966, when I decided I wanted to make an "AIR-CONDITIONED BLANKET".

It could help cool the body, working on the same principle as a room air-conditioner.

My hometown Ambala is known as an important centre for manufacturing of scientific and surgical instruments and workshops of all scales abound. My friend *Bittoo* used to work as a *lathe* mechanic in one such scientific workshop. A couple of years older to me, *Bittoo* shared my enthusiasm for most things outrageous and readily agreed to my proposal to build a small compressor as used in a refrigerator, for my AC blanket. For a prize that was awe-inspiringly mouth-watering - a lunch of endless *chhole-kulche* (Indian stuffed bread with chickpeas curry) at the Bus Stand and *kesar jalebi* (spiral-shaped sweet savoury) at the neighbourhood sweetmeat shop *Manohar Halwai* in Lal Kurti.

Equally fired up, we set out on our mission - *Chalo* (go to) *Delhi* to buy a motor for the compressor!

Much before the break of dawn, *Bittoo* and I were on our way. Even if slightly sleepy, we were a whole lot excited! Walking alongside in our *chappals* we passed the residential *Lal Kurti* (every cantonment has a *Topekhana, Regiment Bazar, Lal Kurti* and *Sadar Bazar*), crossing over the quiet mud fields to reach the Bus Stand. One can normally take the 5 am bus to reach Delhi in 5 hours, ie by 10 am, finish the day's work and set out for Ambala again at 5 pm and get back by 10 pm. Of course, enough trains ply on the Ambala-Delhi route too, but the bus service is just so much more frequent and great for ease of access.

Having finished our 'business' in Delhi, we were back in town. Parking ourselves in a corner of the house, we went to work with the motor, wires and valves - building a small compressor. This we connected to thin but flexible copper pipes that would turn cold, using the same mechanism as a refrigerator.

The outer layer comprised a radiator that was made of flat sheets of aluminium that radiated the warmth. So, the inner layer of the blanket was cold while the outer layer was warm.

The idea was that if the blanket could have a cooling

interior, it shall radiate the hot air outside, so it may be used for cooling the body in the summers while it could be just reversed in the winters – when the hot side would be inside.

The news of our small experiment becoming a success soon spread. Especially with *Bittoo* and I posing together along with a prototype of the "Air Conditioned Blanket" for the news correspondent who came from The Tribune to publish the story of our invention. Meanwhile, *Bittoo* was waiting for his prize - the lunch treat as promised! Much to my relief, father came to the rescue by awarding me a crispy new Rs. 50 note for my invention! And what a wholesome treat it was. At the Bus Stand, we polished off our plates in no time, washing it all down with giant copper glasses of *lassi* (sweetened curd drink)!

The news was published with our picture. As a next step in the course, I applied for a patent.

* * *

The Letter to Jamshetji Tata

Buoyed up with the success of the enterprise, I wrote a letter to Mr. JRD Tata proposing a collaboration with him towards the "commercial exploitation" of my invention.

Still in standard 8, I was super excited when the reply came from the VOLTAS office, asking me to meet the General Manager at Kelvinator, Faridabad.

Straight from school, I boarded the bus to Faridabad. Getting off at the Faridabad bus stand, hitching a *rickshaw* ride, I found myself staring into the face of the guard at the KELVINATOR factory gate.

He asked me who I want to meet. Dressed in my school uniform of a white shirt, *khaki* brown shorts and white keds, I told him that I had been invited by Mr. Tata for a 'collaboration'. And handing him the letter received from Voltas on behalf of JRD Tata, I added,

"I am an inventor. I have invented an AC BLANKET."

In a few minutes, I was peering out of a giant leather armchair in the office of the General Manager - my feet barely touching the ground as I helped myself to the fresh snacks and tea laid out on the table in front of me. The General Manager was amazed at my narration of the idea, and how we'd managed to execute it. At long last, he said he would put the idea to the Company Board, to "look at the market requirements" research data for the same. As I set out to leave, he wished me well and shook my hand warmly.

* * *

The Boy Who Wanted the Sky

My eldest brother was in the Air Force. Posted in Delhi.

Generally spoilt at home, by him I was positively pampered. So, I was naturally delighted to have him back home for the *Diwali* holidays.

At my persistence to buy fireworks, especially *pataakhas*(fire crackers) to celebrate the festival, he took me to the *Pataakha Bazaar* (Fireworks market).

Inside the shop, there were fireworks of all shapes and sizes. The walls of the shop were adorned with colourful sparklers, flowerpots, twinkling stars, rockets, floor *chakkars* (rotating discs) and a spectacular array of fancy crackers. At once enticing.

I insisted I wanted to buy the whole shop of fire crackers and asked the shopkeeper how much would his shop cost. He exchanged glances with my brother, smiled indulgently and commenced to show me some crackers and 'Rockets' so that I may make my purchases.

Now 'Rockets' are my favourite fireworks. And I *sorely* wanted to buy all of the 'Rockets' that were there but it struck me that I needed a sky of my own to fly them.

And for sure, I asked him whether I could buy the sky.

"I **want to buy the sky**, too!" I insisted.

Part II

13

The Making

Chapter 3

EARLY DAYS

As a child, I couldn't have been more spoilt and naughty – getting me to take a bath was nothing short of a daily mission for my mother. And while at it, I would toss and turn, wiggle and twiggle - spraying the water from my curly hair all around, much to my delight and mother's irritation.

Roaming around in the house wearing nothing at all (not even an underwear) seemed the most natural thing to do. But for one day - when my eldest brother and his friends hatched a clever plan.

Catching hold of me, they pinned me to the ground and mock-threatened to cut off my penis, since it goes exposed. The sight of one of them suddenly bringing a knife close to my body and raising it up while it dripped with a bright red liquid, had me bawling my lungs out.

That day onwards, I was never found without my underpants again.

Yet, going to school was an ordeal that I decided I must put up all my forces against. I'd much rather while my days away on the front porch of our house - watching our two Australian Jersey cows, being milked thrice every day, for bucketfuls of milk. I remember how mother sat churning this milk until she retrieved butter from it. And as I planted my arms around her neck, she'd give me some to eat. And of course, I'd run away giggling after I'd stolen some more that I mostly smeared on my face!

*** * ***

Hijacked to School

But they seemed to be relentless in their pursuit to send me to school. In revolt, I would roll over the floor, kicking my hands and legs out into the air while crying copiously. I was quite a handful and amidst my ample shenanigans, my father decided to send me to Delhi to stay with my eldest brother who was a Flight Lieutenant in the Air Force.

One night as I was fast asleep, my eldest brother Chand Bhai picked me up, put me in his lap and took me to Delhi without my knowledge. . . it was not before the next morning that I came to know of having left home in Ambala.

My brother was staying at the Air Force Welsley Road (now Shah Jahan road) Officers' Mess at India Gate, Delhi. In the next few days, I was admitted to the King

Edward Road Children School, on Maulana Azad Road, New Delhi.

Few days into the new school, I discovered, to my great delight - a shop whose display-board read, 'Pure Ghee'. Soon, I started going there, to ask the shopkeeper for *Poori* (deep-fried Indian bread). The shopkeeper would refuse and I would return dejected. But I kept find my way to him day after day to request him for some *Poori* nevertheless, until one fine day, the shopkeeper frustratedly asked me why I thought the shop sold *Poori*. I looked at him and pointed at the shop's display-board on which was written 'Pure Ghee', pronouncing the words slowly as "*Poori Ghee*"in Hindi!

Given my great predilection for *Poori* as a young child, I'd thought the shop sold *poori* made in clarified butter and hoped for it during the half-break daily. The shopkeeper now broke into a gentle smile and explained that it was an advertisement for clarified butter on sale and not *poori*!

Of course, I continued to be just as naughty. The teacher's remarks on my Kindergarten Progress Report card read, "He is very intelligent and given double promotion. Sometimes he is really very naughty in the class". Pulling a prank or being the bully came naturally to me. While playing, fights were common and I mostly ended up beating up some child or the other. Almost everyday, by the time half-break was over, I was invariably found standing, my hands up, facing the wall. Chand Bhai would go straight to the Principal's office to see if I was there, hands up and pressing the wall, standing in punishment. I don't think he ever found me in the classroom when he came to pick me up after school.

Chand Bhai, my eldest brother who's 92 as I write, is a father figure to me and all my siblings. He was firm without being strict, polite without being malleable. Younger to Chand Bhai by a little over a couple of years was Jagdish Bhai who shared Chand Bhai's mess apartment. Jagdish Bhai had a small 10ft x 10ft room on rent in Chawri Bazaar (wholesale market in hardwares in old Delhi) where he would assemble iron parts to make ironing presses (or irons used to remove wrinkles from garments) and sell the assembled irons to buyers or shops in Chawri Bazaar. Jagdish Bhai was handsome in a rugged sort of way and I loved the way he'd fuss over me - taking care to ensure that my bag and clothes were in order for school the next day or getting me to sit down and finish my homework everyday.

And while I knew I was his pet, there was a cause for great consternation for me because of an occasional embarrassment. I loved snuggling up to Jagdish Bhai as he wrapped me in his bear hug, so I'd always sleep in his bed. But there were times when I'd wet the bed in sleep and not be able to look into his eyes the following day. Ashamed at my 7-year old self. For such impropriety.

But Jagdish Bhai never revealed this to anyone. He brought me a solution: Pray to *Hanuman Ji* (Hindu God of Strength and Courage, and devotee of Lord Rama). So, every night, just before retiring, I'd close my eyes tightly, my palms entangled and say, "O *Hanuman Ji*, please take care so I don't wet my bed. PLEASE! PLEASE! PLEASE!"

This worked like magic.

Because on the nights that I forgot to pray, I'd almost certainly wet the bed.

Given this new-found friendship, once *Hanuman Ji* even decided to appear in my dream. A bright red glow glimmering around his head, *Hanuman Ji* was flying, the mountain sitting on his palm, straight at me! Given how mischievous I was, I woke up instantly and started screaming in fear.

The next day, Jagdish Bhai came to rescue. He told me to pray to *Hanuman Ji* and request him: "Please do not come in my dream as I get very scared". And sure enough, *Hanuman Ji* did not show up in my dream. But if I forgot to pray, he was there, without fail.

After a while, I became good friends with *Hanuman Ji* and my faith in him has only strengthened with time. I continue to feel his presence in my life. Most evidently through the countless prayers that he's answered for me.

With Chand Bhai's transfer away from Delhi, it was time for me to return to my hometown Ambala and start school in standard 4.

Now, I had *Hanuman Ji* in my heart and a brand new bicycle as a gift from Chand Bhai by my side.

* * *

Back on Track

Back from Delhi, I was a transformed child. I found myself more sensitive, more conscious and generally more attentive and well-behaved.

This was beginning to show in my class performance where I was beginning to do quite well. I was studying at the Arya Samaj school and especially enjoyed the morning prayer rituals of *havan* and *mantra* chanting.

Inspired by the example of Chand Bhai, I now began to take my younger brother to school. A two and a half years younger to me, Ashwani (Babbi) would ride pillion, one half of his face plastered into the back of my shirt, his little arms running round my tummy.

We were 10 of us - five brothers and five sisters. It was a very unique chain of sibling-nurturing, with Nirmal Didi minding us, after the demise of my mother. Incidentally, we all had a gap of roughly 2.5 years amongst us.

First came, Chand Bhai (with whom I share my birthday and who's daughter is younger to me by 2 years),

Then, Jagdish Bhai
Then, Kanta Didi
Then, Mohan Bhai
Then, Nirmal Didi
Then, Sharda Di (just 'Sharda' after a while!)
Then Guddi
Then Kukku
Then ME
And finally, Babbi.

I remember mother was pregnant with Babbi at the time of Chand Bhai's wedding. While this may seem incredible today, such things were quite common then.

Older to me by twenty two years, Chand Bhai married when I was about 2.5 years old. I still remember it had been raining heavily through out the day of his wedding and my father was busy entertaining the numerous guests and visitors.

But come rain or shine, father used to invariably take me out 'for a walk' in his lap every evening. So, around the customary time, I began to cry to be taken out for a stroll. And despite all the goings-on, father gathered me in his arms and out we went, under a big black umbrella even as the skies poured.

I had just finished my standard IV examinations when my mother expired.

Chapter 4

WINDS OF CHANGE

In those days, Standards IX and X were considered the two most important grades of a pupil's academic life. Simply put, Matriculation (Standard/Class X) was a big deal. It was the exam that would 'open the doors' to a career path of choice. So, Chand Bhai got me admitted to DAV School, which, back in the day, was considered the best school in Ambala.

When I started Grade X, our Headmaster Puran Chand, commonly known as *Headmaster Saab,*taught us English Now, *Headmaster Saab ,* a particularly tall man with wheatish complexion, dressed in his stark white *kurta pyjama* and grey waistcoat, sporting a Nehruvian *topi* (cap), had a particular eccentricity of manner that made for great mirth among the students, but to which he was largely oblivious. During his lecture, he would continuously scratch the palm of his hand, the frequency increasing as he went deeper into the lecture. He never imagined that each time his back was turned to us, that boys would imitate his action - the whole class noiselessly dissolving into peals of laughter in welcome relief from boredom. But one day, I was caught laughing. *Headmaster Saab* asked me to standup and tell him the reason for the sudden mirth, failing which he would suspend me from the school.

I told him we were copying him - scratch his palm, absent-mindedly. This infuriated *Headmaster Saab*- he made the entire class stand up on the bench and put up our hands. As he came round with his cane to rap us on the knuckles. I don't think any of us ever forgot this bashing. Some of the boys even got blue marks on their knuckles from the cane. It was hurtful, to say the least. Everybody was unhappy but nobody had the guts to say anything to his face.

The next morning, a few boys from our class stood outside the school main gate - shouting the slogan *'Headmaster Murdabaad!(Death to the Headmaster!)'* and stopping other students from entering the school. After an hour, when nobody went through the school gates, the peon came out. He was told that all the students were on strike and refused to enter the school premises. He went back in and possibly informed this to the Headmaster.

Soon,*Headmaster Saab* came out, his white *pyjama* riding up his calves as he walked towards us, cane in hand. A cold stupefying shiver seemed to run down our central nervous systems. He stopped and stood silently before us. Eyes moving from one boy to the next, as we lowered our gazes. Suddenly, the first row of the boys who were leading the slogans, went inside the school without a word. Everyone else followed suit. We filed into the school, a disciplined queue of quiet boys. The strike was called off. Nobody ever spoke about it again.

As I progressed from one grade to the next, my performance steadily improved. And I began to find myself taking my academic pursuit seriously. Perhaps a decent indication of my achievements at this time was the appearance of my name on the Honours Board of my school for ranking *IInd* in the Class X (Matriculation) exams in Ambala.

***

Master Numericals!

After DAV High School, Ambala, I secured admission at DAV College Jalandhar for my pre-University. Situated just outside the city and spread over several hundred acres of landscape, the sprawling college campus bore the semblance of a University, with its two hostels, each containing a few hundred rooms, dozens of mess and massive building 'blocks' dedicated to each individual subject such as Chemistry, Physics, Botany, Zoology, etc.

In more ways than one, DAV College was a premier institution. It was a matter of pride to be from DAV College, Jalandhar. The kind of school or college you go to, leaves a mark on your personality and character. And I may say that my college has left an indelible stamp on mine.

While DAV College was widely reputed as the best college in the whole of Punjab, Haryana and Himachal taken together, it secured a whole new dimension every year. Roll no. 1 of every class ranked first in the Punjab University: be that pre-Medical, Bachelor's in Science or any subject in Arts.

Arranged in order of 'merit', my roll no. was 337 when I joined pre-University (Medical) at DAV College. I was put in Section B1, while roll numbers started from 301, denoting the top students in descending order.

I think, with conviction now, that the DAV College system made it almost certain that I study, to the best of my abilities.

There were 2 hostels in DAV College Jalandhar: LR Hostel and Meher Chand Hostel for Seniors. My hostel, LR Hostel was an almost 300 metres long, C-shaped two-storey building (with 300 rooms in every block!).

Our hostel gates used to close at 9 pm sharp. In the unfortunate situation that one was late, the boy wasn't allowed to enter the hostel without registering his name in the "LATE COMERS" Register. Every 'late-comer' was required to report to the Warden the following evening . . . who would then call the parents and inform them of the same. Naturally, we were all really scared of the Warden and actively avoided a late entry.

Now, the guard on night duty had another task - he used to strike an hourly siren before going around to wake up the boys. He kept a register where we used to write our names and room numbers, every evening. Some boys wanted to wake up at 4 am, others at 3 am or still others at 2 am. The guard would go around like a human alarm-bell, waking up each one according to the time as mentioned by him in the register.

This was an especially useful facility for the boys in the LR Hostel 'Scholar Block', widely touted as the Block where boys 'study throughout the night' in the balcony. Not entirely without truth. Every evening, all the students in the Scholar Block would sit and study here, in this massive balcony that overlooked all our rooms. As a boarder in the 'Scholar Block' (I was in Room no. 212 on the first floor), I could easily remember the exact number of square concrete slabs that made up the balcony floor. There was always competition (quite literally!) about who studied till the latest into the night. The 'Scholar Block' moniker was also perhaps earned by virtue of the toilets. Walk into any of them and till date, you shouldn't be surprised to find solved Physics numericals on the walls down to the lavatory floor!

The campus atmosphere was so charged with academic discipline that it was natural for us to be obsessed with 'ranks' 24x7. We were thinking, discussing and working towards bettering our performances all the time. The class exams' results were displayed on the Notice Board for all to see, so while we knew where each one stood in class but more importantly, it acted as the catalyst that inspired greater dedicated effort at improving individual performance each time.

We used to have Special Classes every morning starting at 7am and two practicals every Sunday (one in the morning and another in the post-lunch session)! One could reach out to any Professor at any time for guidance. In hindsight, it strikes me now that everything was geared towards nurturing an environment that rewarded scholarship. We had an excellent library that was open 24/7 and never was there a book that couldn't be found therein. The reading experience was made especially richer with the free stationary and the many 'rounds' of steaming hot tea that were brought in earthen *kulhads* (baked clay cups) free of charge. There was a liberal supply of paper and pens for use by scholars and on cold evenings, one could go and sit close to the heater while studying. Should one still feel the lunch break and walking past the Admin Office and the Principal's office, turning to find the mammoth 'Biology Block' to your left when the Principal's voice pours into your ears through the microphone to state the *Thought of the Day.* Turn right towards the 'Chemistry block', and you might hear him mentioning the new college rules and discipline-related matters such as punishments for miscreants, late comers etc. By the time, you can trace your steps to the 'Physics block' on the backside, chances are that you are listening to the names of the topper students who've aced their class tests and the coveted prize of being able to approach teachers of choice.

At the time, DAV College was especially known as the breeding ground of the best scholars. For several years consecutively, all of the first ten rank holders in the University exams were from DAV. It was a no-brainer that Punjab University's topper was ALWAYS a DAV-ite, without exception. Even the authors of syllabus bestsellers were invariably teachers of our college (all our teachers, especially the Heads of the Departments had written course books on their respective subjects, that were referred to widely). Or the first boy of DAV College, the previous year.

Which brings me to Ramesh Bansal.

After a few weeks of starting college, I met Ramesh Bansal - a brilliant scholar in my Block who held the record of acing every exam that he sat for. Bansal did not just achieve the first rank in the exam, but he positively quashed all previous records in Punjab University by far.

A simple middle-class guy with wheatish complexion who walked with a limp because of the Polio that affected his childhood, Bansal was considered a legend. Each year he passed a grade, he would write a textbook - his "Class notes" were very popular among the students, and everybody had them. Book publishers would literally queue up to buy his class-notes and publish the same. Every year, 'Ramesh Bansal Class Notes' sold like hot cakes.

When I first heard about him, I was naturally curious to meet him. I knew that he taught students in his spare time, possibly to supplement his family's income. But never did I dream that he'd offer to teach me Physics.

At Rs. 10 a month, I was slightly hard-pressed. I knew I could spare between Rs 8-9, but you don't bargain when Ramesh Bansal offers to teach you. So, I agreed to his offer. Every other evening, we went for a walk to the canal which was about 2 km on GT Road. On the way, he would ask me Physics Numericals, challenging me to solve them mentally! Where earlier I'd been utterly scared of them, now I gradually began to enjoy solving them.

That year, Bansal wrote his most celebrated textbook "Master Numericals to Master Physics".

As for me, I secured distinction marks in Physics, this increased my score and percentage, in turn pushing up my rank to 312 (against the 337 when I'd joined). I overtook 25 boys to emerge really close to the top spot. Most importantly, I came to be known as 'Master Numericals', a title my classmates bestowed on me for my ease with Physics numericals and the sheer joy at every opportunity to solve them!

Part III

The Breaking

Chapter 5

THE FALL

I was back home in Ambala after my Class XI, for pre-Medical. This is when I happened to meet Master Tara Chand, Vice Principal at SD College (Ambala Cantonment) and a good friend of my father's.

He pressed upon my father to admit me to SD College - offering free books, free milk during lunch time at the college canteen and free tuition from any teacher. He also offered a cent percent waiver of tuition fees. A lucrative offer. Plus the attraction of being so near home. The damage was complete. Instead of going back to DAV College Jalandhar, I found myself walking in through the gates of SD College Ambala.

Here, conversations revolved around movies, girls, and boys and girls. Exciting, entertaining, even enlightening.And sure enough, I was distracted.

I hardly paid any attention to classwork. Lectures were dull and not half as lively as to what I was being exposed to outside the classroom. Consequently, my class performance suffered and I just somehow managed to scrape my way through the end-term exam. But the blow came with mefailing to make it to Medical College Rohtak by 1%! And as if to reinforce the lesson, I failed to make it to CMC Ludhiana by a few marks. Yet again.

Remorse gradually gave way to despondency. An education in Medicine was now a distant dream. I managed an admission in the GMN College, Ambala Cantonment for a B.Sc (Bachelor's in Science) degree. I'd so pathetically duped myself of securing a seat at a Medical College, that I gradually slipped into a casual comatose back-bencher. Days were frittered away in casual gossip.

Those days, *Rajesh Khanna* movies were the rage. I remember imitating his style of walk and talk. Even started sporting *kurtas* (loose collarless shirts especially popular in the Asian sub-continent) like those he wore. I wore my hair long and styled on the side with waves carefully grazing the temple. I also began to jam in college, playing the Mandolin.

I imagine those days were enjoyable, but not content. I was a hippie with little hope. Looking to find the right pair of boots to go with my bell bottoms.

Not a day passed when I did not repent my decision to not return to DAV Jalandhar. And the subsequent failure at acquiring an education in Medicine.

After a few months (somewhere in the early 1970s), things took a turn. It was one of those sultry afternoons when the land is parched and you look out of the window to check for the remotest likelihood of rain. My eldest brother was back in town and told me he has some 'news' for me after lunch.

So, I was waiting for him on the front porch of our house where our ancient *Neem* trees rustled endlessly, bringing in a comforting breeze. Chand Bhai joined me shortly. His hair had visible strands of grey now but he looked just as handsome as ever. Gently wrapping a friendly arm around my shoulder, he told me that our cousin Dr L R Aggarwal, a Professor at the Mahatma Gandhi Memorial (MGM) Medical College, Jamshedpur had informed him that a few 'seats' from the *Waiting list* had just become available for new admission.

My eyes widened and then realising the import of what he'd just said, they welled up. I hugged Chand Bhai for a long time. That afternoon, I was the happiest soul if there ever was one.

Our cousin was Professor and Head of the ENT (Ears, Nose and Throat) Department at the Tata Main Hospital, Tatanagar in Jamshedpur. He'd studied at the same college as Chand Bhai and was his junior by a couple of years. At the time, he'd stayed with us in Ambala and our families had continued to be close.

Dotted with numerous clubs, golf courses and pretty gardens, Jamshedpur is a clean and green city. Peaceful and beautiful - unlike any other major city in India. As a senior doctor, his quarters were very well appointed. Spread over 2 acres, the bungalow was surrounded by a massive garden. The front lawn was perfectly manicured with a lovely rose garden and a golf putting green. On the backside, was a huge kitchen garden that grew everything from brinjals to cauliflowers and bananas to mangoes. I stayed with him at this incredible villa-like facility which also housed a separate outhouse complex with 5 servant quarters and a *dhobi ghat*(an especially appointed place with ample supply of water where clothes are washed by hand) .

As all the doctors working at the Tata Main Hospital

resided in quarters within a single huge complex of bungalows, most of my classmates were sons and daughters of renowned doctors such as Anita Khosla, Srirekha Reddy, Sheeba Marcos and lived close by. All of them, including my cousin, were members of the very elite Beldih club and so it was a pretty robust social circle with frequent 'catching-ups' among fellow doctors at the Golf course or a movie at the amphitheatre once a week or so. During this time, I made friends with Rakesh Sahni and Rajesh Loomba; and those friendships have lasted a lifetime. Rakesh, handsome and sparkly, back from an English schooling in London, was an eloquent and expressive speaker. He had a way of charming his way into your heart with an infectious laugh and a mischievous wink. Loomba (don't remember ever calling him 'Rajesh'!), on the other hand, was this fair, handsome, soft spoken and sober young man - like the one in the really old English movies. The one who doesn't speak much but is most often heard. The three of us were a riot, our distinct personalities easy foils to each other. After finishing work at the campus, the three of us would often go to the nearby Bistupur (market in Jamshedpur city centre).

All was going well. Except that Bihar was extremely strike-prone those days, often directly impacting students' lives. One of our classmates, K.K. Singh who stayed at the 'Mango Hostel' used to actually lead the strikes (he continues to be a close friend). A complete shutdown of college meant that our coursework suffered and we were constantly pushed behind time. For instance, the one and a half year long first professional MBBS course took almost two and a half years to complete.

Strikes occurred every few weeks if not earlier. In such times of indeterminate and abrupt college closures, we could not stay at the hostel and would mostly leave for our hometowns. Before long, of course, we made better use of our time and the student concession tickets. Instead of taking the train back home, we once went to Benaras (now Varanasi), Bombay (now Mumbai) and other places.

Now while the strikes were indefinite in terms of time duration, they were almost certain in the matter of occurrence. And calculating backwards when exams were first postponed in our 'First year', where we lost a 1.5 year, thereby finishing the First year in roughly 3 years; it was evident that our 4.5 years MBBS degree would take anything around 6 - 7 years, by modest estimates!

In view of these circumstances, all three of us - Rajesh, Rakesh and I decided that we needed to immigrate to whichever Medical College we could find a seat at.

Luckily, Loomba managed to migrate to Rajendra Medical College, Patiala while Rakesh shifted to Dayanand Medical College, Ludhiana. I found a new home too, at the HP Medical College, Shimla. However, we continue to remain very much in touch till date.

* * *

A Few Pegs of Chilled Shimla Evenings!

Formerly known as Snowdown because of its location in the Snowdown area of Lakkar Bazaar in Shimla, the HP Medical College is a state-owned Medical College and Hospital in Shimla in the state of Himachal Pradesh. It was here that I first delved in clinical research work.

The hands-on clinical research exposure helped me

gather diverse research inferences and write several papers that were published in both Indian and international Science journals. Sometimes, I'd even add my friends' names on request!

Guiding me through this process was the unassumingly friendly, exceptionally bright and soothingly soft-spoken supervisor, Prof. D S Puri. The Head of the Medicine Department at HP Medical College, Prof. Puri was an excellent clinician and teacher. Of a slender frame, kindly demeanour and scant appetite (except for his love for a drink every evening!), we'd often wonder if he survived on air. It was his willing support (painstakingly editing, cleaning up and formalising) and constant encouragement that enthused me to write and publish very many research papers in my time here.

Here, I had the great opportunity to work on several research projects simultaneously. All of the following and many other research works were published and presented at various conferences by my Supervisor Prof Puri and me. Except for the last one.

-- Cleido cranial dysostosis - in a family of 8 persons (it is a congenital defect where the frontal cranial bone does not fuse and there is a soft portion in front of the forehead - also the patient is able to bring together both shoulders as the clavicles are missing)

– Effect of rarification of oxygen on right side of heart and its reflection in ECG (t I did this project in Lahaul and Spiti where due to the high altitude, the air is severely low on oxygen)

– Effect on RNA and DNA on Gastric Juice in Peptic Ulcer (Blind study using2 agents and 1 antacid in patients of peptic ulcer)

-- Incidence of Sexually Transmitted Diseases in people living in monasteries in Himalayas (surprisingly

CYSTICERCOSIS IN AN ENDEMIC PROPORTION
IN A VILLAGE IN HIMACHAL PRADESH.

BY

Dr. A.K. Aggarwal [1]

Dr. L.S. Pal [2]

Dr. H.K. Sarin [3]

&

Dr. D.S. Puri [4]

Departments of Medicine and Radiology,
H.P.Medical College and Snowdon Hospital,
Simla-171001 (H.P.)

·—

1. Assistant Physician, Department of Medicine.

2. Resident Medical Officer, Department of Medicine.

3. Professor & Head of Radiology Department.

4. Professor & Head of Medicine Department.

Address for correspondence:

Dr. D.S. Puri,
Professor & Head of Medicine Department,
H.P.Medical College,
SIMLA-171001 (H.P.)

A New-found Passion: Writing Scientific Research Papers
One amongst many - "Cysticercosis in an Endemic Proportion
in a Village in Himachal Pradesh"

Cysticercosis, which is produced by pork tape worm, Taenia
solium, has a world wide distribution with special prevalence in
countries where raw or undercooked pork is eaten(France & Ponce,1974[6]
and Plorde, 1977[12]). Besides India & far east the disease has been
well described from Southern Italy, Portugal, South Africa and South
America (Bickerstaff,1955)[2] . Even in countries where cysticercosis
is prevalent the disorder has been described either as isolated
case reports or collection of such cases of over a period of years.
We had the opportunity to come across seven cases of cysticercosis
in a small village having a total population of only 37 situated
in a hilly terrain in Himachal Pradesh. The study of these cases
forms the basis of this communication, as cysticercosis in an
endemic proportion in a small community has never been reported as
yet.

MATERIAL & METHODS

A 45 years old male, native of a small village at an
altitude of 1720 meters above mean sea level in the interior of
Himachal Pradesh was admitted to Snowdon Hospital attached to H.P.
Medical College, Simla with the history of fits. Besides clinical
examination,detailed radiologic and serologic investigations were
undertaken. Histopathologic examination of the material obtained by
biopsy of one of the subcutaneous nodules established that cysticercosis was responsible for generalised seizures in this individual.
History from the patient revealed that his brother and a few other
natives of his village were also suffering from same type of fits.
All the suspected persons were brought to Snowdon Hospital,Simla for
detailed work up. Following investigations were undertaken :-

1. Radiologic examination of skull, spine,chest,shoulder and
   pelvic girdles and legs.

2. Complement fixation test for cysticercosis.

3. 12 lead Electrocardiogram.

4. Biopsy of one of the subcutaneous nodules, if present.

OBSERVATIONS AND RESULTS

Out of 37 adults studied, seven cases belonging to both sexes revealed evidence of cysticercosis. The age of these patients ranged from 19-54 years. The distribution of patients according to age is shown in table I.

TABLE I

The clinical presentation of these cases is shown in Table II

TABLE II

RADIOLOGIC FINDINGS

Out of seven cases, calcified cysticerci in the pelvic girdle and calf muscles were visualised in 5 (Fig.I) while in shoulder girdle in 4 cases (Fig.2). Evidence of calcified cysticerci in the skull as well as spine was not found in any of the cases.

COMPLEMENT FIXATION TEST was positive in 4 cases (1:16) and negative in the rest of the cases.

12 LEAD ELECTROCARDIOGRAM : was normal in 4 cases while 2 cases had generalised T wave inversion and one case had complete left bundle branch block pattern(Fig. 3).

HISTOPATHOLOGIC EXAMINATION of the biopsy specimen of the sub-cutaneous nodules was undertaken in 3 cases and in all of them it revealed presence of cysticercous cysts (Fig. 4).

DISCUSSION

Cysticercosis cellulosae, the systemic form of the infection with larvae of the pork tape worm, is an uncommon condition in man, as the larval stage generally develops in the pig. However the cysticercosis stage of Taenia solium is found in man occasionally. Human

infection occurs when ingested or activated endogenous ova of
this parasite release larvae, which pierce the intestinal wall and
enter the blood stream. The common sites of localisation are the
nervous system, skeletal muscles and subcutaneous tissues. Occasionally
the heart, lung and peritoneum may also be involved (Arseni &
Samitca,1957[1] and Obrador, 1948[10]). Cysticercosis, being an uncommon
condition in man has only been described in isolated reports from
the different parts of the world, particularly where raw or undercooked pork is eaten. We observed seven cases suffering from
cysticercosis in natives of a small village situated in difficult
hilly terrain. The detection of these seven cases out of 37 natives
implies that 18.9% of the total population was suffering from
cysticercosis. The occurance of cysticercosis in such an endemic
proportion has not been reported so far. The high incidence of this
disease in the population of this village is attributed to the custom
of eating uncooked pork at the time of local fairs, and festivals and
religious congregations. Due to difficult terrain, lack of means of
communication and illitracy this custom has prevailed in this
particular village for years. Of these seven cases of cysticercosis
five had features of involvement of the nervous system, two had
palpable nodules only and one had nodules in addition to the recurrent
meningoencephalitis. This case finally developed mental changes and
committed suicide. Varied manifestations like epilepsy, hydrocephalous,
mental changes, meningoencephalitis, partial or complete blindness
due to deposition of cysts in the optic disc and paraplegia have
been reported due to cysticercosis(Vijayan et al, 1977[15] ;Hoffmans &
Guthrie,1975[7] , Singh et al, 1966[14] , Lombardo and Mateos, 1961[9], and
Cabieses, et al 1959[3] and Dixon & Lipscomb, 1961[5]). In our cases
epilepsy and recurrent meningoencephalitis without any signs of
raised intracranial tension were observed in 5 cases. The presence
of subcutaneous nodules was of considerable help in diagnosis as it

was discovered in 3 cases though some authors have stated that
they are too infrequent to be of much help in the diagnosis
(Schnur & Richardson, 1977 [13]).

Calcified cysticerci were found in the pelvic girdle
muscles and calf muscles in 5 cases (71%) and in the shoulder
girdle muscle in 4 cases (57%). Radiologic studies were of
immense help in diagnosis, though according to some authors
(Schnur & Richardson, 1977 [13]) calcified cysticerci are of limited
value in diagnosis. Skiagrams of the skull & spine did not
reveal any calcified cysticerci for it is well known that the
incidence of calcification of cysts deposited in the brain is
infrequent and it may take years before they get calcified
(Wilcocks & Menson-Bahr, 1972 [16]) .

Complement fixation test was positive (1:16) in 4 and
negative in the rest of the 3 cases (Powell et al(1966) [11] have
reported that serologic studies notably haematologic and complement
fixation tests are both sensitive and specific in most of the cases
but recent studies appear to refute this conclusion. [8] It is,
therefore, not surprising that 3 of our cases inspite of definite
diagnosis of cysticercosis had negative complement fixation tests.

Although cysticercosis commonly involves the nervous tissue
skeletal muscles and subcutaneous tissue, [4] rarely involvement of
heart has been reported. In one of our cases the presence of left
bundle branch block in the absence of any other aetiology suggests
that deposition of cysticercus cyst in the course of left bundle
produced this electrocardiographic abnormality. Complete heart block
due to deposition of cysticerci in the bundle of His has been
occasionally reported (Wilcocks & Menson-Bahr,1972 [16]). Since the
detection of these cases the villagers have been educated regarding
the hazards of eating raw or undercooked pork and people have left
this custom which had been prevailing in that community for decades.

SUMMARY

Cysticercosis cellulosae, the systemic form of
infection with the larvae of the Taenia solium is an uncommon
condition in man. Seven cases of cysticercosis in a small
village situated in a difficult hilly terrain have been reported
in this study. The clinical presentation were grandmal
epilepsy (4 cases), recurrent meningoencephalitis with
subcutaneous nodules(1 case) and subcutaneous nodules only
(2 cases). The presence of subcutaneous nodules and calcified
cysticerci were of great help in the diagnosis. Diffuse
myocarditis as evidenced by generalised T wave inversion in
all 12 leads was detected in two cases. Complete left bundle
branch block due to deposition of cyst in the course of left h
bundle was seen in one case. Complement fixation test was
positive in 4 cases (57%). Cysticercosis in an endemic proportion
amounting to public health problem in a small community has not
been reported earlier in the literature.

REFERENCES

1. Arseni, C. and Samitca, D.C., Cysticercosis of the brain.
   Brit.Med.J.,2:494, 1957.

2. Bickerstaff, E.R., Cerebral cysticercosis; common but unfamiliar
   manifestations. Brit. Med. J., 1: 1055, 1955.

3. Cabieses, F., Vallenas, S.M. and Landa, R.J., Cysticercosis
   of the spinal cord. Neurosurgery, 16; 337, 1959.

4. Case records of the Massachusetts General Hospital, weekly
   clinicopathological exercises. Case 40-1977, New Eng. J. of
   Med. 297(14): 773, 1977.

5. Dixon, H.B.F. and Lipscomb, P.M. (1961) cited by Singh, A.,
   Aggarwal, V.D., Malhotra K.C. and Puri, D.S.; Spinal cysticercosis
   with paraplegia., Brit. Med. J., 2: 684, 1967.

6. France-Ponce, J., Neurocysticercosis, Neurology: Proceedings of
   the tenth international congress on neurology, Barcelona, Spain.
   September 8-15, 1973. edited by Subirana,A. Espadela, J.M.,
   New York, American Elsevier, 1974, p. 234-250.

7. Hoffman, S.F. and Guthrie, T.H. Jr., Cerebral cysticercosis,
   South Med. J.., 68: 105, 1975.

8. Kagan, I.G. and Norman, L., Serodiagnosis of parasitic diseases;
   Manual of Clinical Immunology, Edited by Rose, N.R., Friedman,H.,
   Washington, D.C., Amer. Soc. of Microbiol., 1976 p.382-409.

9. Lombardo, L. and Mateos, J.H., Cerebral cysticercosis in Mexico.,
   Neurology (Minneap); 11: 824, 1961.

10. Obrador, S., Clinical aspects of cerebral cysticercosis.
    Arch. Neurol. Psych. 59; 457, 1948.

11. Powell, S.J., Proctor, E.M., Wilmot, A.J. et al: Neurological
    complications of cysticercosis in Africans: a Clinical and
    serologic study. Ann. of Trop. Med. Parasitol. 60: 159, 1966.

12. Florde, J.J., Cestodes (Tapeworms) infections. Harrisons
    Principles of Internal Medicine. Mc Graw Hill Kogakusha Ltd;
    Tokyo, Japan.Edn. 1977. p. 1113-1115.

13. Schmur, J.A. and Richardson, E.P. Jr., Progressive dementia
    and Seizure disorder in a 62 year old native of Cape Verde
    Islands., New Eng. J.Med., 297: 773, 1977.

14. Spinal cysticercosis Singh, A., Aggarwal, N.D., Malhotra, K.C.
    and Puri, D.S.; Spinal cysticercosis with paraplegia.,Brit.
    Med. J. 2: 684, 1967.

15. Vijayan, G.P., Suri, M.L., Sahai, B. and Singh, M.; Periodic
    lateralised discharges in E.E.G. in cerebral cysticercosis.
    Neurol. India, 25: 38, 1977.

16. Wilcocks, C. and Manson-Bahr, P.E.C., Manson's Tropical
    Diseases published by Bailliere-Tindall, London. Edition 1972,
    p. 340.

<u>TABLE I</u>

<u>Showing age distribution of cases.</u>

<u>Age in years</u>	<u>No. of cases</u>
15-24	1
25-34	2
35-44	3
45-54	1

<u>TABLE II</u>

<u>Showing clinical presentation of cases.</u>

<u>Clinical presentation</u>	<u>No. of cases</u>
Grandmal Epilepsy	4
Subcutaneous nodules	2
Recurrent meningoencephalitis with subcutaneous nodules.	1

incidence was a full 100 percent here!).

While the research data from the Himalayan monasteries revealed extremely worrying positive samples, it was the one study that could not be published because of the ultra sensitive nature of the information.

I passed MBBS in 1975. And my bonding with Dr. Puri especially strengthened during my Internship, followed by the two House Jobs I did under his supervision. It was based on an easy and unaffected friendship that developed in the process of a dedicated collaboration over many a research project that now extends well beyond the clinical laboratories and medical wards.

Every day at 5 pm, after the internship, Professor Puri would wait for me at the college gates. We'd walk together to the Shimla Mall. Now, this also happened to be my regular meet-up point with Ninni and Vinnie, my buddies from GMN College (Ambala Cantonment) where we were studying together for the B.Sc degree before I got admission in MGM Medical College Jamshedpur. Narinder Garg (Ninni to us) was a happy-go-lucky guy, the kind who loves the good life and is generally high- spirited. The last, quite literally - as there was never a day in the week when we did not all sit down together for a drink!

Vinnie (Vinod Garg) had just joined his family business in timber. Vinnie's family were known as the 'Timber Kings' because they were the largest foresters in Himachal Pradesh. A famous timber trail in Parwanu also belonged to them, and Asia Tawi Jammu was one of their first hotels. Vinnie and I were especially close. And for the longest time, Vinnie's brother wanted me to marry his sister-in-law.

Both Ninni and Vinnie took to Professor Puri and he to them, like fish does to water. So, it was a jolly group of four every evening at the Mall, Shimla. Professor and Ninni were members of the Shimla Club, so we'd mostly park ourselves there or alternatively, at the Oberoi Clark's. Some evenings, we'd go to Vinnie's house, the Timber House (adjacent to St. Edward School in Shimla). For a casual change of scene, my room at the YMCA (Young Men's Christian Association) sufficed. The very memory of those evenings spent together every single day of the week warms the heart. As did those full bottles of Scotch that one of us would invariably get. Ninni, of course drowned half of it! Vinnie following close, consuming a quarter. The quarter remaining was Professor's. I pitched in for what they'd jokingly call "a spoonful".

The memory of those warm evenings spent amongst a close circle of friend s still melts my heart.

* * *

Finding Her

While visiting Vinnie at his home, I often came across Vinnie's charismatic elder brother Yash Pal Garg or YP to us. Older to Vinnie by some 10 years, Yash (of the 'Timber Kings' fame) was a very flamboyant businessman, hotelier and forester. Sometimes, if we were around, he'd invite Vinnie and me for a drink and chat in the evening.

One Saturday afternoon, when the three of us were lounging in their drawing room, Yash asked me about my 'plans' for marriage. I was a little taken aback at the suddenness of the inquiry but I didn't let it show.

I agreed it was indeed the right age for me to consider marriage. "However, since my income is low - I would like to marry a doctor girl if possible", my response was candid.

YP said, "In a class of 40 boys, there may be, at the most, 10 girls . . . So, by your logic, only 10 boys shall get to marry doctor girls. Shall the rest all stay unmarried?" Yash was a very persuasive and focussed businessman. He had a metaphorical way of speaking where he'd ordinarily start with a question and then gradually reveal his mind to the audience.

"I am not so unlucky, I hope," I averred, wondering where this was going.

Without further ado, YP said, "I want to propose a girl for you."

While Vinnie and I sat listening in rapt attention, YP continued, "She is my *saali* (wife's younger sister). She has just completed B.Ed (Bachelor's in Education) and is a teacher. And she hopes to continue teaching after marriage."

I told him once again that I did not, at all, intend to marry a teaching girl.

Yash, however, was not one to be easily dissuaded. He insisted that I meet her together with his wife (i.e. the girl's elder sister) at the Mall. I was totally against this idea because saying 'NO' would become even more difficult once the meeting took place. And in all probability, I would stand to lose my friendship with Vinnie.

So, I tried to reason with him. I said, "You are rich… your wife is obviously rich, too…If I get married to your wife's sister, she will end up being the wife of a poor doctor, while her elder sister is the wife to a super-rich business tycoon."

I continued, my argumentative skills at their best, "Your wife may have several loads of money to spend, while my wife will never have enough, at least in comparison. Very soon, she will develop an inferiority complex, before slipping into depression eventually."

Yash insisted that I should treat him like my elder brother, and said, "Oh! I want to hear none of this! And leave your financial limitations and problems to me. I will take care of them."

But I knew better. I couldn't expect another to support me financially, because it begins as a small gesture and before long, snow balls into something else that leads to misunderstandings and an eventual fallout, especially amongst the closest relatives or friends. Besides, I did not want a strained relationship with my friend Vinnie so I was firm in my refusal of his proposal without being impolite.

Not one to give up easily, YP went to meet my father in Ambala and presented his case. My father was easy. He said, "It's Arvind's decision entirely. If it's a 'Yes' from him, it's a 'Yes' from me And vice versa. I've left it to him. And I wouldn't want to pressurise him in any way."

So, I started looking for a girl for myself. My eldest brother Chand Bhai, who was 'responsible' for conducting the matchmaking for all our sisters, used to find prospective alliances through matrimonial columns in the Hindustan Times news daily. I had seen him through the entire process starting from writing the 'Bio data' to putting out the advertisement and conducting the matrimonial correspondence.

My sister Sharda and my brother-in-law used to live in Kasumpti, near *Chotta* Shimla. So, I used to visit her every weekend or whenever I had a day off from the Medical College, Shimla. A prime attraction were the fluffy *parathas* (Indian fried bread) she'd serve me with the lip - smacking *gobhi-shalgam achaar* (cauliflower-turnip pickle) that she made herself. Just as she'd placed the steaming *parathas* on my plate, over them would land a fat dollop of white butter - something I so utterly loved.

One day, I put out the advertisement in the Hindustan Times, with my sister Sharda and brother in law's address and phone number.

Those days, advertisers would often use a Post Box no. on the advertisement, this number helped the news paper office to receive the responses on behalf of the advertiser and send in a weekly batch of the responses received.

I'd taken the plunge.

Soon, a neat brown packet of envelopes started coming into my sister's house every week. Sharda would telephone me to inform of the packet's arrival and I would come down during the weekend. Laying out the envelopes on the bed, we would make our choices and I would write to the prospective parents-in-law under my brother in law's name, enclosing my full bio-data.

Of all the correspondences, there were two girls who really interested me. One was a doctor from Rajouri Garden, Delhi. Her name was R. Jain.

It was a middle class family like mine. Her father was a doctor and so was her elder sister. A day was mutually decided for the first family meeting and Chand Bhai, Sharda, my brother-in-law and I went to Delhi.

As we walked into their house, everywhere I looked - there was the doubtlessly dominant presence of a pervasive shade of dark bottle green. All the rooms of the house, even the balcony ceiling were painted in this one uniform shade of deep dark green. The furniture was really old and again green in colour. Even the dining table and its chairs were painted the same colour. The only contrast was perhaps the grey of the cold granite floor against which my bare feet rested, a tad uneasy. They ate their dinner at 7 pm, like a traditional Jain family.

At the earliest opportunity that I found her seated near me, I told her quietly, my eyes to the ground (to make it appear real!), thatI already liked someone but my parents were forcing me to look for a match of their choice. I also told her, quite unscrupulously, that my folks were expecting a big fat dowry, given that 'Doctors fetch a good market value' and this I think really helped put an almost immediate end to the matter.

The other proposal was of a Doctor (then doing House job in Paediatrics) from Chennai. Her parents were in the manufacture and export of garments. I'd already sent my picture and particulars under my brother in law's name but there had been no response. Weeks went by, then one day my brother-in-law received a call from the girl's eldest brother, an ex-Major - Indian Army, who'd switched over to the family's export business. He informed us that his parents and his sister (the prospective match!) were coming to Himachal to arrange the engagement of her younger sister in Solan, and had plans to visit Shimla and 'see the boy' if possible.

Back in the day, it was conventional for the boy to go, see the girl for a prospective matrimonial alliance, not the other way round. But there were not many North Indian families in Chennai, so people usually travelled up north to look for prospective alliances.

One Sunday afternoon, while I was casually hanging around the house at my sister's, a car pulled up. And a middle-aged man emerged to ask for my brother-in-law. He said that his son had telephoned us and he was here from Chennai to fix a time for meeting.

After chatting with my brother-in-law for a while, he revealed that his wife and daughter were waiting in the car downstairs and proposed that we meet on a mutually convenient date at a restaurant or so, 'for the *boy* and *girl* to meet more comfortably'.

My brother-in-law, however, insisted that they come up instead of waiting in the car and enjoy cups of fresh Himalayan tea with us. Casting aside all protocols of formality, we went down to invite them in.

It was then that her mother and she walked into the house. *She* was tall, slim, bright-eyed and wearing a *sari*. *She* was carrying her *sari* very well.

For the next 3 hours, her father and I talked about my recent trips to Leh, Ladakh and Kinnaur; as I narrated some of my strange encounters while conducting the medical camps.

Chapter 6

STORIES FROM THE CAMP

Story 1: The Gompas in Ladakh and Leh

I returned to the Medical College with some of the most spectacular coloured stones with inscribed *mantras*, that I picked up outside the *Gompas* (Tibetan Buddhist monasteries) in Leh.

In Leh-Ladakh, the *Gompas* abound. It is customary for both men and women to live in there together. These men and women are mostly unmarried.

As a part of our medical research project, I went therein to conduct ECG of the people staying in the *Gompa* I also did their pulmonary capacity test and blood test. And I acquired test samples from some 200 persons of both genders.

After returning to my camp, I gave the blood samples to the Pathology lab for regular investigation including test for Sexually transmitted diseases (STDs).

Soon after, the shocked technician called me to ask where I had procured "such samples". He suspected that I may have used a contaminated syringe as every one of the samples tested STD positive!

We decided that I shall go back to bring fresh samples from the *Gompa* once again. So, the very next day, I went to the same *Gompa* to procure the samples again, tactfully. We found them all to be positive, again. This time, I revealed these results to my supervisor Prof. Puri. He was similarly excited but advised against the inclusion of sensitive details in my research report.

Later, I wrote a paper titled 'Effect of Rarification of Oxygen in High Altitudes on Heart and its Reflection on ECG'. This paper was published in the API or Association of Physicians of India Journal.

I looked around. I realised her father and mother had been listening to me without blinking. My sister and brother-in-law, too. I looked at *her*, our eyes meeting briefly, for the first time. Meena.

* * *

Story 2: The Precarious Pass of Rohtang

Amongst my many experiences in the Himalayas, there was one particularly exciting adventure that befell us as we travelled from Shimla to Kinnaur across the Rohtang Pass to hold our medical camp.

Our caravan comprising a truck, a bus and 4 jeeps started from the Snowdon Hospital and Medical College Shimla in the wee hours of the morning. I resolved to travel by the new jeep, thinking it would be a different experience. And sure it was - a very different experience, in more ways than one.

It was a brand new Mahindra jeep. But the moment we started going uphill, the jeep's engine developed a snag. It began to heat up and we could smell something burning.

Glad with our early detection of the problem especially because we had a really long journey ahead of us in terrains that were precariously steep; we went back to the Hospital for a replacement. This time, the next jeep - another brand new Mahindra, travelled uphill for quite some time. Yet, before long, the engine began to heat up. So, we decided to take it easy and go slow the rest of the way, in the process managing to lose touch with the rest of our caravan who'd already driven ahead.

We continued to drive until we reached Sunder Nagar. Here, the construction of the Beas Satluj Link Project was underway. The purpose was to divert some water from Beas into Satluj to increase the storing capacity of Bhakra Dam (or Gobindsagar dam) for generating electricity.

As we drove through the construction site, I saw an incredible sight. The road in front of us by which we were approaching Sundernagar, toppled in a massive landslide. Momentarily, the entire land mass of rocks and boulders and soil just fell through. Immediately turning back our jeep, we managed to escape the landslide by a whisker.

The roads would be closed now with no hope of travel until the next day. It was imminently important to find a shelter for the night. This was a challenge because all the other vehicles on that road were similarly stranded and everyone was thinking the same thing as us. Nightfalls in the mountains are especially tricky - suddenly plunging you in such pitch darkness that the sense of desolation and danger is very real. Dusk would fall any moment now and that would mean a desperate situation.

We decided to find out the nearest PWD Guest House, if there was any. With directions from a few kind locals, we found ourselves at a PWD facility and luckily for us, the rooms were available. We took two rooms for the four of us. Then, we asked the guard-cum-cook-cum-caretaker to bring us some chicken and cook dinner, gently pushing a few currency notes into his palms. He smiled sheepishly, looked at his palms and promised us some local wine, too.

Next morning, we rose early and found that all the rooms were taken. People had come in during the night and checked in. The guard informed us that the road had been cleared and it was ready for vehicular movement. So, we left the guesthouse and went back to Sunder Nagar, and by afternoon we'd reached Kullu.

Here, the first thing we decided to do was surrender our jeep to the Medical Superintendent, Kullu. The vehicle, in its present condition, would not be able to climb the steep Rohtang Pass and we needed to make an alternate arrangement.

Our caravan and we had now been separated for over 24 hours (since the landslide last afternoon) and there was no hope of finding institutional help. We were now on our own.

We took the local bus and reached Manali.Here, we found a truck driver who was about to ferry some goods across Rohtang. So, we requested him to take us across the Pass, too. He agreed, but he said he would go only later that night. We agreed to that.

We waited until it was time to leave. But now he had some bad news for us. The owner of the truck had arrived and would now travel by the same truck, and given the fully loaded cargo, he did not have space to accommodate all of us.

So, we spoke with the truck owner. What we now agreed to was the closest I've ever come to insanity. While two of us could be accommodated inside the driver's cabin alongside the truck driver and owner, the other two of us would 'sleep' on the roof of the driver's cabin - I, being one of the two.

The truck started. The two of us lay opposite each other, our legs stacked against the head of the other. The temperature was beyond freezing, hovering around a minus 30 degrees centigrade. But we felt thankful that we were dressed adequately. Besides, the truck driver had kindly given us a blanket to cover ourselves. But what did we know?

With the first acceleration of the truck, the wind seemed to have jolted us out of the truck. The two of us squeezed ourselves tightly into the crevices of the truck's roof, holding on to this one blanket. But what made it especially difficult was that the ends of the blanket would part on either my side or his, and the chilly mountain air would gush in. We were already frozen, but I think that night I heard my teeth chatter away while my fingers went numb, in a way I hadn't known earlier.

Just before one reaches the top of Rohtang, there is a flat area called *Dhalli*. *Dhalli* is a resting place and it is usual to find a *Dhalli* at many places in Himachal.

We spotted a small roadside motel on this *Dhalli*. By now, we were cold, hungry and as near dead as it's possible for alive men to be. So, a dinner of lentil soup, rice and mutton sounded like a dream from distant lands.

Interestingly, we learnt that many shepherds bring out their cattle to graze on these hilly terrains. They don't mostly have money, so as they pass through these small motels - they will occasionally exchange a goat for food.

The motel owners will then kill the goat and bury it in the snow which is in plenty; taking out the animal, in parts, to cook. So mutton was cheaper and mostly easy to find around these places.

We climbed down the truck and had our dinner here. And never has a meal tasted so delicious to me ever before.

We discovered that they were renting a cot with a pillow for half a rupee per night. This was very cheap, even by 'those days' standards. I got myself a cot, took off my shoes, slipped them under the bed and fell fast asleep.

In the morning, my shoes were gone! And the sight was outright scary. As I tried to look for my shoes under the bed, where I'd left them the previous night, I saw that my cot was supported on four pieces of stone and there was a deep hole under the cot. Had I seen it before going to bed, I wouldn't have been able to sleep at all.

With my shoes now gone in the hole, I could only hop around barefoot. Our truck was parked about 100 meters away from the motel but there was snow everywhere.

I desperately needed to find something to wear on my feet because the ice cold ground was beginning to bite and would knock them numb soon. The motel owner came to the rescue. He gave me pieces of gunny bag to tie around my feet and two pieces of plastic to help wrap them to keep them from getting wet.

Hopping and skipping, I somehow managed to reach the truck.

Climbing up Rohtang was scary. For most of the time, our truck was literally tilted backwards at 30 degrees. The steep slippery roads with sharp hairpin bends were so narrow that we dared not look down lest we get a heart attack.

Reaching atop Rohtang, we saw a display-board that stated *'Satluj starts here.'* We stopped the vehicle. The sight was breathtakingly beautiful. And I think we appreciated the place more because we were alive.It was a once-in-a-lifetime adventure that made us realise that it's an entirely different world up there on the hills, especially on the Rohtang Pass.

It was around mid-day, the next day, when we reached our destination. Here we met the rest of our Camp team.

I think they were more relieved than happy to see us. They had been much too anxious for our news. Since the last two days, there had been regular announcements over the radio. Air Force helicopters had been directed to fly low in their 'look-out' for us. The apprehension that we'd met with an accident was rife. Nobody could, atfirst, believe that we were back or the kind of incredible ride we hitched.

However, the mountain drivers are extremely adept at their art and habitual with regard to its practice. They drive on roads so narrow that the front and rear tyres on one side of the vehicle are oftentimes 'outside' the road, seemingly hanging in the air. And the skill of the drivers is a wonder of itself. Our driver could see the truck coming from the opposite direction even from a distance when none of us could. They are conversant in their language of horns, dippers, etc. At times, I felt that our driver was talking to the roads, the trees and the traffic as it passed by. This is their world. Like an alternative world. Like the world under water.

I looked up. My brother-in -law, sister Sharda and *she* smiled happily.

* * *

Story 3: How many fathers?

To see the starting point of the Satluj, to see how people crossed the river Satluj sitting on a trolley that they pulled themselves over a rope, left a deep impression upon my mind about the hills and the deep influence they have on the lives of the people around them.

The lives and rituals of ordinary men and women were deeply interesting to me.

One day, I had a strange encounter. A middle-aged man of medium build, wearing a long robe tied at the waist, walked into my campclinic. His name was Ramesh Lal Thakur.

During the course of recording patient history, I asked him,

"What's your father's name?"

He asked,

"Which father?"

I did not know what to say. I was too afraid to ask, *How many fathers you have?*

He was a strong man. And I guessed if he took to violence, I would be a poor match. Besides, it might especially hurt given the cold climes. So, I held my peace and heard him as he continued to speak.

After a few minutes, I asked him again.

"What's your father's name?"

He replied,

"Just now, I asked you *Which father?*"

I did not know what to say. I asked him, very innocently, "What do you mean ? I don't understand . . ."

He looked at me. Then, he went on to explain.

"I have 3 fathers . . .", he continued,
"Eldest. Sohan Lal Thakur
Second. Ram Lal Thakur
Youngest. Ghanshyam Lal Thakur."
I did not quite understand. "How can you have 3 fathers?" I asked incredulously.

"Just like in Mahabharata, the five Pandava brothers had one wife ...same way," he replied matter-of-factly.

My curiosity was now piqued. I really wanted to know more about this man but could not quite bring myself to ask another question.

A few weeks later, this concept became clearer to me when we went to Kinnaur to conduct a medical camp.

On the hills, they have large parcels of land. It is neither easy nor practical to return home every evening after work as there is no transport and one may have to walk 20 - 30 miles one-way to return home. Besides, it gets dark suddenly and quickly. So, the men build a small cottage on the land and stay there after work. Once a week, they come home.

Now, the woman who the eldest brother marries becomes wife to all his brothers. They come home in turns and sleep with her. Just outside the room, a big nail is placed on which the brother who's inside the room will hang his coat and cap . . . this indicates the house is 'full'.

This woman is wife to the men in the family and all children are from her. None of the children will ever know the biological father. So, they will *all* have *all* fathers.

With regard to rights regarding property, all the children will have equal share in the joint property of all their fathers. Interestingly, there's no fight over property because the male children, too, will grow up to have one wife, . . . and common children. Hence, property passes from one generation to another without division.

As for their sisters, they ask for her preference over which portion of the land she would like to have and give her her equal share in the property. But the best part is that she is given that piece of land which she selects.

On her marriage, the sister will take away this share that she has selected and the lady they marry, will bring her own share. So, the size of the property continues to, more or less, remain the same. This is a very natural mode of keeping the property from division.

Speaking of marriage, I also learnt another strange ritual. In each of their homes, the family will isolate a room. On the roof of this room, they will carve a hole. This is the toilet.

All family members go to the roof of this room to relieve themselves. Faeces accumulates in this room for years together. Until the time the daughter in the family gets married. At the time of her marriage, they open the room, take out all the faeces which has, over the years transformed into manure, and spread it over the land parcel she selects. This is their dowry system.

My prospective father-in-law and mother-in-law sat listening in rapt attention. I could see that my audience was waiting for more stories. And I didn't disappoint.

* * *

Story 4: Of Angoori

On the two banks of the Satluj, there are two quaint little villages called *Chotta* (small) Ribah and *Bada* (big) Ribah, well-known for the mushrooming of wineries. For good reason, too. The abundant quantity of grapes that grows on this soil, is particularly rich in quality and responsible for the singularly nuanced taste of the locally-brewed *Angoori* (wine).

In fact, most locals brew their wine at home. A rudimentary formation of an indigenous brewery is often found parked in the basement of the house. Locally sourced grapes are boiled here, the vapours condensed and collected in a kettle-like utensil. The first distillation product is 'mild' grade and mostly used by females and children while the second or third distil is much stronger and customarily offered to guests or men.

The strength of the alcohol is unpredictable because there is no way to measure the potency of the indigenous produce, differing by its method and degree of production from house to house. But it's universally accepted (by all who have sampled it) that despite its various degrees, *Angoori* remains one of the purest concoctions made from the best grade of grapes. In fact, it tastes better than the French white wine but due to the unfortunate lack of organised marketing, it has remained largely unknown to the taste buds of the world.

Incidentally, the villagers mostly will not have corks to secure the locally-brewed liquor bottle's mouth. So what do they do? They take a frozen piece of butter, place it on the mouth of the bottle and hit it with their fist. The butter goes in, seals off the mouth of the bottle, acting as a cork. Cheers!

Every household in this area customarily has 3 floors: basement for storing the animal fodder. This storehouse is necessary because these areas remain cut off from the mainland, sometimes over the course of 6 - 9 months in a year because of the heavy snowfall, losing all access to food or other essential items except for certain emergency supplies that may be reached through the helicopters.

In fact, every house has a door each on the ground floor and the first floor for entering or exiting the house. In the snowladen 6-9 months when the ground floor door is jammed, people use the first floor to exit the house on the street or to enter the house.

The top floor comprises bedrooms for guests and visitors while the ground floor will usually comprise the living quarters for the family. The bedrooms, the kitchen, washrooms will all be here.

Given the close proximity to China, a large number of the families are practising Buddhists. So, it is customary for the family with 3 sons, say, to send the eldest son to the monastery to be a monk. The second would get into business and the youngest would be a teacher.

Both men and women wear a thick woollen robe known as *Chonga*(a long, loose garment resembling a *Kaftan* or a *Phiran* worn by Kashmiri men and women). Like the Kashmiris, they hold a warm earthen pot containing hot coal known as *Kaangrj* close to their abdomen, inside their *Chonga* Effective in keeping their bodies warm in the sub-zero temperatures, this earthen pot is called *Kaangri* and is used by men, women and children. It reminds me of Shimla where we normally used hot water bottles (made of rubber) during patient examination to warm our hands so that patients don't wince at the sudden shock of the cold touch. In fact, almost all doctors carry these hot water bottles while conducting their 'rounds'.

During the 15 days of my stay on the river bank, I was hosted by the family of Swaroop Seth, one the *most important* persons in the area whose family ran the largest grocery shop in the village.

And I discovered the functioning of the site was particularly interesting. Right outside the shop, near the gate they'd put a wire where the customers could hang their shopping lists.

During the day, 3 - 4 men would help pack the requested items, labelling them and placing them in a basket, each with a scribbling that mentioned the total due amount for payment by the customer.

A day or two before the appointed day every week, when everybody's groceries were ready for delivery, they would go around the village, announcing through the loudspeaker - the date, day and time for the collection of their groceries.

The payment list was displayed outside the shop in advance. On the appointed day, the customers would queue up at the store to make their payments and collect their supplies.

Swaroop Seth's connections in the plains from where he used to arrange the bulk transportation of food grains and other groceries by trucks helped render his store the only grocery shop in the region, catering to several villages. He was a hands-on grocer, conducting daily 'rounds' to inspect the activities at the store. On his *paalki*.

It was quite a sight. Twice a day, Seth would be ferried to the store (from his living quarters on the floor above) and back, on the *paalki* (palanquin). At the store, the *paalki* doubled up for this elaborate chair with maroon cushions and pink velvet rugs, all securely held together with coir ropes, on which Swaroop sat ensconced. And then I realised - it was his home-grown solution to replace a wheelchair!

Those days, there were no electric wheelchairs. I found out that Seth used to be a state-level sportsperson when he lost the use of his lower limbs in an unfortunate accident on the hills. But his mind continued to be agile and he quickly made use of his connections to earn a livelihood by setting up the grocery store for the villagers. Seth continued to be regarded widely for his services. And for his generosity.

A few days before my clinic ended, I bought from the store - some raw almonds, cashew nuts and *chilgoze* (pine nuts) of a quality I'd not seen earlier. When I went to make my payment, the storekeeper handed me a neatly packed 2 kg gunny bag containing my goods, refusing to accept the cash. Stitched over the gunny bag was a neat little hand-written note which read,

" Thank you for your medical services! Please visit again. With compliments, Swaroop."

It's amazing how through our memories, we travel to faraway lands, reminiscing over episodes that remain etched on our hearts. Forever.

It seemed as if time had stopped. But it hadn't.

It was almost 3 hours that everyone around me had been keenly listening to the narrative. I paused and my brother-in-law gently gestured to Sharada to get refreshments for the guests. And as if on cue, sitting on the tea tray were little bowls of almonds, cashew nuts and *chilgoze.*

Chapter 7

SHIFTING GEARS

Back to routine. Evenings at Shimla Mall with friends. And conducting clinical research by the day. I was back at work and super busy. By now, my hands were full of research projects and 1 was churning out one research paper after another. By the time I was around 27, I already had a record number of scientific paper publications to my name.

At times, my senior colleagues would request me to add their names as co-authors. Publications were considered vital while applying for higher education because they are seen as a mark of solemn scholarship and academic rigour . At times, I used to oblige them. But the same was not always possible. Before long, envy creeped in. Principal Mehrotra's unit, that year, was unable to publish any research while I, with guidance from Dr. Puri, had put out 4 scientific papers.

Pettiness paved the way for my transfer from Medical College, Shimla to a remote village dispensary in Kotbeja.

Kotbeja is a little village, about 3000-4000 ft. below Kasauli. A small dispensary had just been started there, in fulfilment of an electoral campaign promise.

The nearest accommodation was the PWD Guest House in Kasauli, where I put up for the night to join the dispensary the next day.

The morning after, my compounder came to pick me up from the PWD. It was a one and half hour walk down the hill through crooked and slippery stone paths that seemed to give way with every step. There was no way to reach the village except on foot.

As we made our way down the steep descent to the dispensary, I began to sweat profusely until I took off my tie. After a while, my coat came off, and by the time I managed to climb down all of the 4000 ft. descent to the dispensary, my sweater and shirt were all off.

The dispensary was a stark room - about 10 ft x 20ft, only one half of it covered by the roof. There wasn't much furniture except for a table and one rickety chair plus two small stools. There was no fixture where the seat of the chair was, so a narrow wooden plank had been strategically placed to function as a seat. A couple of buffaloes were tied outside the dispensary to graze, probably by some local villagers.

A compounder, peon and a medical officer (me) comprised the staff of the place. The three of us waited the whole day but not a single patient walked in. The room was sparse and there wasn't even the basic supply of medicines. After a while, I thought I would send the peon to get a few essential medicines. He informed me he would bring the medicines but return only the next day because of the long distance to and fro. Besides, I saw no reason for his immediate return.

In the evening, it started to rain. There was no way to go back to the PWD now as the ascent was dangerously steep and slippery. I asked the compounder if there was any place where I could stay the night. He looked at me, and then looked around.

I realised that the half-room dispensary was converted into his bedroom at night. He offered me to sleep with him. We shared the one small cot he brought out from the corner. For dinner, we boiled some rice. Then, he added in some salt and *jeera* (cumin seeds). We shared the meal, sitting cross-legged on the bare ground.

Sometime during the course of that evening, I asked him, "In a place like this, how do you manage to spend your time? There are no patients, no place to stay, nothing to eat . . . nobody to talk to."

He told me that he stayed here for 15 days and went home for the remaining 15 days every month. While returning from home, he would bring some rice and other basic grocery like sugar, tea, some vegetable oil and kerosene oil etc. Interestingly, in the 15 days the compounder was home, the peon would double up for the compounder. When the compounder returned after 15 days, it was the peon's turn to go home.

So, every month each of the two was home for 15 days each, returning to relieve the other. Of course, there was no vigilance, no visitors, not even patients.

At the end of the month, the compounder made a trip to the District Hospital to collect the salaries for both of them - this was the existing arrangement.

Now that I'd joined, I thought we might split into 3 shifts of 10 days each.

But they had a different proposal for me. They told me they would manage as they were doing then. I may stay home for all 30 days.

I could do my 'practice' at home and come at the end of month to collect the salaries for all three. Handing them their salaries, I could return home. Repeat the process every month. This seemed to be a convenient enough arrangement and I did this for 2 months.

Until one day, my father, who continuously saw me loitering around the house, asked me if I had been kicked out of the job since I was always home.

I told him the story. He exclaimed, "You will forget all the Medicine! It's better you resign immediately from the job and start your clinic here."

That's how I gave up my job and started practice in Ambala.

On hindsight, the experience revealed to me, from close quarters, how our healthcare system was plagued with rather morbid 'conditions' of inaccessibility, unavailability and lack of standardisation. And I began to think of creating a system which could smoothen the bumpy road to healthcare delivery for the remotest person on the last mile.

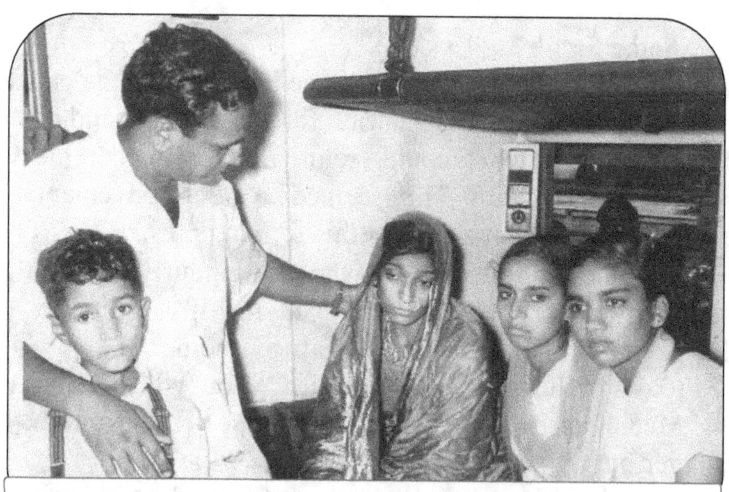

At my sister Kanta's Vidaai (post wedding home-leaving ceremony) In picture. Standing: My brother Jagdish and Myself (as a young boy). Sitting (L to R): My sister Kanta (bride), my third sister Sharda, Jagdish Bhai's fiancee Bimla

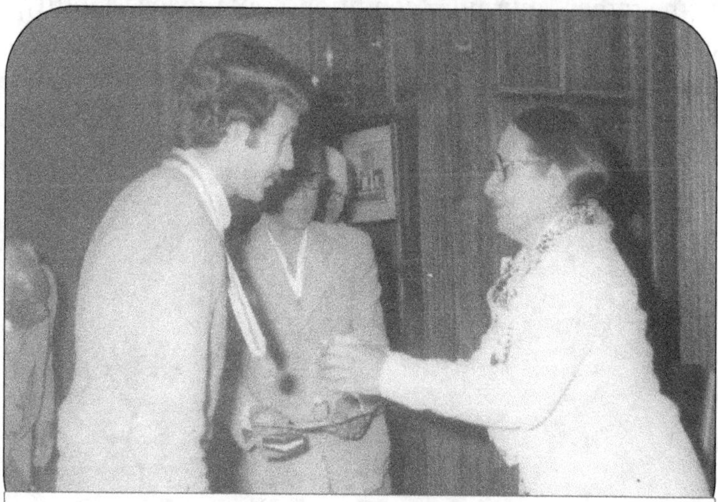

Receiving the Governor's Medal from the Governor (Himachal Pradesh) for making a record number of blood donations

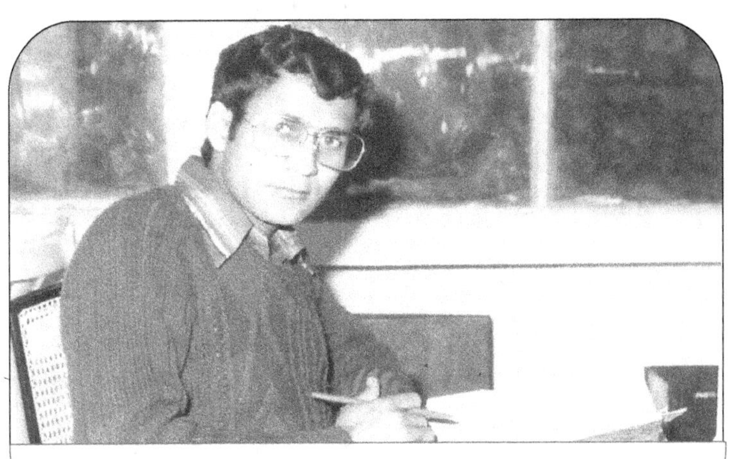

In my room at the LR Hostel "Scholar Block",
DAV College Jalandhar

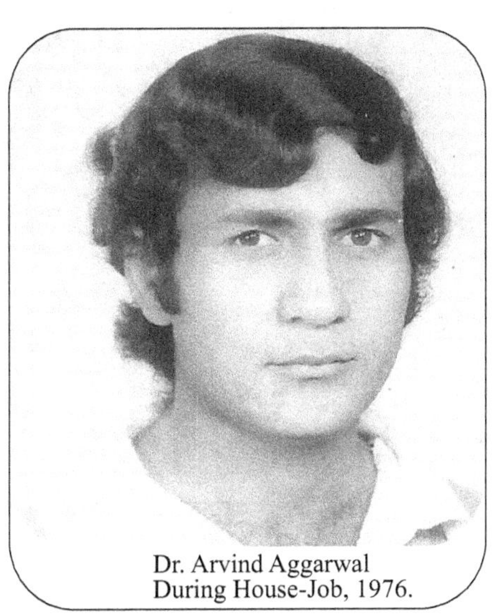

Dr. Arvind Aggarwal
During House-Job, 1976.

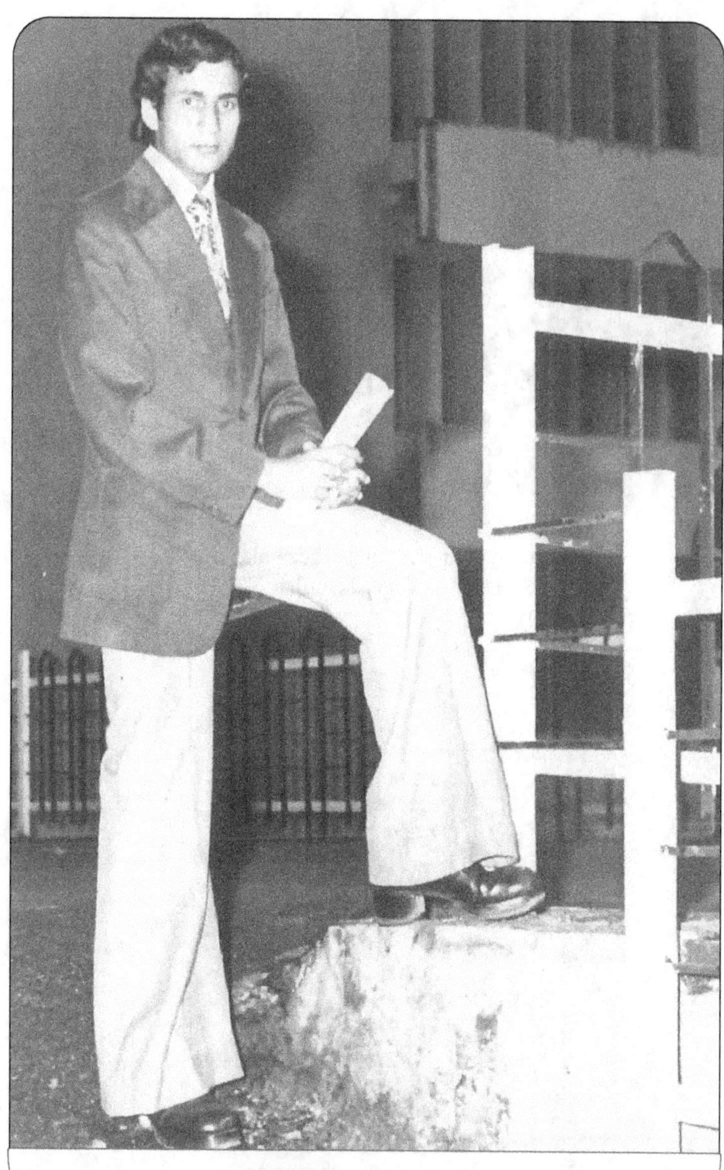

Zindagi ik safar hai suhaana, . .
Sporting long hair and bell bottoms, my Rajesh Khanna avtaar

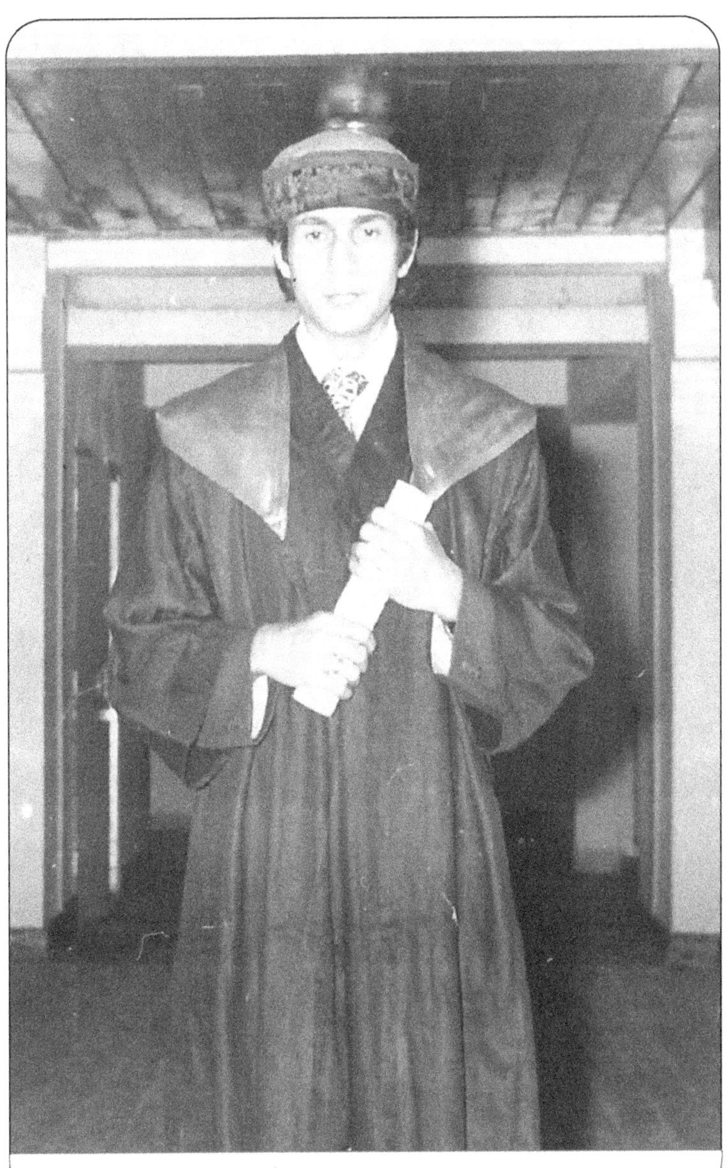

After: Convocation - HP Medical College, Shimla
Here I am!

Part IV

Flying Out

Chapter 8

MEENA

Except for a few sentences in the course of the narration, I hadn't really spoken to her when she'd visited us with her parents. But in my mind, I could see her walking into the house, carrying her *sari* confidently about her.

That evening just as they were about to leave, her father had said to my brother-in-law, "We have approved the boy. Let us know your decision". He promised to call the next morning at 9 am.

After they left, there was no further discussion on the topic. Sharda, brother-in-law and I had continued to sit around the table and chat up about the 'camp experiences'.

But the next morning, dot at 9, he called. And we

hadn't really thought about it. So, when my brother-in-law, the exposed telephone receiver in one hand, asked me, *"Abbe Saale!* (Oh, brother-in law!) Now what should I say?" (Note: Although used endearingly in this context, the Hindi colloquial equivalent for brother-in-law *'Saale'* is most often used as a common swear word), I instantly replied,

"Okay, say *Yes!"*

In the *'What's next?'* phase of the negotiated marriage, a couple of months passed during which there was no communication.

Then, one day my brother-in-law received a letter from the girl's brother asking him to "send the boy to Chennai for a few days as the girl wants to talk to him".

Now, I did not have any leave from the Medical College to go to Chennai. Besides, I did not wish to put myself in an awkward situation where I may be under duress to make a decision. So, we communicated my inability to travel right then, instead proposing for them to come over.

A few days later, they messaged that they would be coming to Chandigarh shortly. And we agreed to join them in Chandigarh for a second meeting.

This time, my father joined us from Ambala. My brother-in-law and I came down the same day from Shimla to meet them.

She had come with her parents. She expressed her desire to speak to me alone. When we were by ourselves, she told me she had a medical issue. Ever since birth, she had a visible swelling on her right leg and this she did not want to hide from me. She showed me her leg and asked me to ask her all questions that came to my mind, but first as a doctor and then, as a prospective suitor. That was Meena.

I looked at the tests and reports that she'd brought.

They were all normal. I made photocopies of these and asked her for a couple of days.

Taking them to Shimla with me, I intended to show them to Prof. Puri for his opinion, but I stopped short.

I liked and appreciated Meena's candidness. Frankly, she need not have risked revealing it to me. On the other hand, she did not want to hide it lest it became an 'issue' later.

It was a childhood disease that was neither affecting the heart's functioning nor the kidneys. So, I needed to take it in the right spirit. Besides, Meena's frankness had bought me over. *What if she had not revealed this, in the first place? I would have come to know only later.. but what could I have done then . . .?*

I did not want to punish her for her sincerity. I took my decision, without discussing it with either Prof. Puri or anybody else. And because of this decision, I've got myself 42 years (at the time of writing this book) of blissful togetherness and still counting.

(By the grace of God, all is well since our marriage in 1980. While resting, Meena needs to keep her right leg slightly raised by placing a pillow under her leg. She is very fond of short dresses and shorts; and regrets, at times, not being able to wear them to her heart's content! But that's hardly a thing).

My friends from Shimla , of course, made a spectacularly grand *baarat* (marriage procession from the groom's side) at the wedding. My memories of Vinnie and Ninni dancing remain one of the most animate expressions of our wedding.

Vinnie arranged to bring all our friends from Shimla to Almora. On the way, he picked up even a *dhol waala* (a local drum player) from Panchkula in his second jeep that had just about enough space, after all those crates of whisky and soda.

In fact, Vinnie gifted us our memorable honeymoon, return tickets to Jammu and Srinagar from Chandigarh and reserved for us the special Presidential suite in his family hotel *Jammu Asia Tawi* Those were the most awesome two days of our new life together.

When we entered the hotel, the hotel staff was lined up to receive us. The rituals of welcoming newly-weds, replete with a round copper plate with a little earthen lamp, flowers and vermilion were all in order. Once each of our foreheads were touched horizontally with vermilion, the staff wheeled in this giant-size cake decorated with a dancing couple in a glass ball that read *'Happy Married Life!'*

Our honeymoon suite had a lovely bed showered with rose petals. And the refrigerator in the room was full of chocolates and wine! For lunch the next day, Vinnie invited us home and in the evening, there was a musical 'Jagjit-Chitra Night' at the hotel. The whole of Jammu Kashmir cabinet was present that evening and we were there as his special guests.

Back from our honeymoon, we were invited to my in-law's place for the marriage reception. So, Meena and I left for Chennai.

Gupta Garments - owned, managed and run by my in-laws, was widely regarded as something of a pioneer in garment exports from India.

Their residence was the entire first floor of this sprawling mansion on a total land area of some 10000 square yards while their factory was on the ground floor. I noticed that the factory workers, some 300 of them, were mostly Chennai-based or from the nearby villages. A lot of women worked on the factory floor, with most of them working barefoot. They lived very simply. While eating their food (that they brought from home in steel lunchboxes), they would use their fingers as forks to eat rice with a sour soup called *rasam.* They would not touch the glass to their lips while drinking water. Afterwards, they would carefully wash the utensils and put them away into their bags.

It was almost a fortnight that we'd been in Chennai, and still there was no Reception. I felt particularly awkward as they were all so busy, it seemed nobody had any time to plan our Reception.

After a couple of months passed and yet there was no talk of a Reception date, it felt as if I was just waiting there indefinitely. One fine morning, I took up the task of directly asking my father-in-law,

"Do you have a date in mind for the Reception? Or maybe I should come back later . . .", I suggested.

Funnily enough, almost immediately everything was organised and the Reception was held. I realised that the reason for delay in holding the Reception was linked with their plans of setting up a nursing home for me, settling us in Chennai and soon.

However, I wished no such thing. And soon after our Reception, we returned to Ambala. I had, by this time, already quit my job after having been posted at the Kotbeja dispensary, near Kasauli.

Now, I dived headlong into my private practice. It was very hard work at first, with patients walking in at all hours. As the word spread and my clinic became busy, I found myself working through the weekends too.

With time, we started doing well in practice. But Ambala is a small town and Meena was not happy here. Meena's parents ran a huge factory in Chennai employing some three hundred workers. The factory set-up was contained within their residence which was a huge mansion spread over thousands of square metres. In contrast, our house was a very modest, middle class establishment in the small town of Ambala. Meena wanted to go abroad and make a better future for us.

* * *

The Switch!

The time that we spent in Chennai soon after our marriage had revealed to me the world of global business in the garment industry. Within the family, I was especially inspired by Meena's eldest brother, the globe-trotter Dr. Surinder Kumar Gupta. He held an MBBS from the Armed Forces Medical College, Pune; but he'd shifted gears to move full time into garment exports after leaving the Army and was doing very well. At that time in the early 1980s, he'd travelled half the world twice over. Attracted to the garment business, especially its unique opportunities for global travel, I decided to make a switch. My in-laws' business included quite a large volume of exports to Swedish and the European markets. So they suggested that they open an office for us in Sweden with permission from the Reserve Bank of India (RBI). But we would first need to go to Chennai to "learn the ropes".

This would mean that Meena and I would go to Sweden and handle business with their big retail chain customers such as H & M and others. And this was precisely what we wanted! We agreed and as suggested, we moved to Chennai for a few weeks to learn all about garment exports, especially the production and manufacture of garments.

Days graduated into months. Like any other employee, I was now spending my days working in the factory and office. Several months passed, still there was no sign of opening an office in Sweden or even any plan for the same.

Finally, one day I put my foot down, and just like last time, went ahead and asked my father-in-law about his plans for us. It transpired that they'd applied to the RBI for permission. In fact, they'd made two applications for two offices, one in Sweden for Meena and another in Germany for Neena (my sister-in-law). But sanction was received for only one of them - the Germany office. RBI had refused to sanction permission for a second office in Sweden, and they did not know how to break the news to me. Unflinchingly, I asked him, "What are the options?"

He said, "Go back to your profession. Both of you are doctors. We can even set up a good nursing home for you where-ever you wish."

In fact, he wanted us to set up shop in Panchkula, then a new upcoming township near Chandigarh and bought a plot for the same.

But I'd invested a significant amount of my time and efforts in the factory. I'd left my medical practice in Ambala to come here and learn this new business of garment manufacture and export. And I wasn't about to just turn around and leave. I hoped to travel the world and build a business. On my own, if need be.

We decided to open a garment factory in Delhi. We started with a very small fabrication unit in Delhi where we were doing sub-contract work for my in-laws for the initial couple of years.

And then one fine day, my two brothers-in-law parted ways, each of them setting up separate factories. The word-mark GUPTA GARMENTS (an established name in Chennai) was retained by my younger brother-in-law Kaku Gupta (or Varinder Kumar Gupta) for handling buyers in UK, France (Carel) and Australia (Kala Craft).

My elder brother-in-law, Dr. S K Gupta set up a new factory by the name GUPTA & COMPANY to handle the German buyers and the very well-known large Swedish retail chain by the name of Hennes and Mauritz, commonly known as H & M.

It was, more or less, a clean divide in business, because each brother was already handling his three most important customers, at the time of the partition. All was well.

Except that we suddenly found ourselves stranded. No one now wanted to pass us the fabrication work as earlier.

Left to our own means, we started from scratch.

But we had neither the know-how nor any access to the foreign or export market. Except that in 1981, the year my daughter Shilpi was born in Chennai, we considered it most lucky that immediately after her birth, I went for my first maiden trip to Japan for a Trade Fair. (I'd never been abroad before. Shilpi's birth brought us joy as we'd never known earlier).

Without the requisite market experience or finance, we ended up doing petty work for the domestic market.

With great difficulty, I managed an entry in Taj Hotel's in-house boutique *Khazana* Manufacturing for a boutique is tricky, the quantities are very small and the variety really large, with many different styles. And especially luxe designer boutiques such as the Taj's showcase only a select and limited quantity to ensure exclusiveness of style, thereby pushing up production costs. Besides, the payments were mostly delayed and that posed a problem as I was expected to pay staff salaries and labour charges regularly. So I was actively looking for an alternate buyer when one day I saw a *'Call for Tender'* advertisement in the papers: Uttar Pradesh (UP) State Handloom Corporation was looking for a contractor to make shirts for their 100 plus showrooms pan-India.

At the time, I already had some experience making shirts for established brand names such as *Taj Khazana* and *Snow-White* So, I submitted their products manufactured by me as samples to apply for the tender. On the appointed day, I went to Kanpur for the 'Tender opening'.

There were about 7 - 8 participants including me, but the others were all locally based. After submitting our tenders, we were waiting out side the General Manager's office, who would soon 'open' tender.

The waiting area had ample sofas, chairs, a central wooden table which held some magazines and a couple of the day's papers. It was a well-lit space and I took my place on one corner of the sofa that allowed me ready access to the reading material. As I casually flipped through one of the magazines, one of the other applicants approached me and inquired about where I came from and my line of business. I told him my experience. He then left my side after telling me about the 'hostile work environment' of the place. Moral of the story: I stood no chance and I should go back.

Then there was this other person in a grey bush-shirt and a grey beard who said he had direct access to the General Manager and that the latter had already called him before the tender announcement. He informed us of having sent 5 big cartons of 12 whisky bottles to the General Manager's house earlier in the day. I realised that everyone had a different story to tell and they were, in fact, very creatively engaged in dissuading me from participating in the tender. I kept listening to them and was genuinely amused at some of the stories. As we waited, the peon came and announced my name, saying that I had been called in. Suddenly, one of the storytellers rushed forward and holding the peon by his collar, shrieked into his ears, "And what should we do?"

The peon said timidly, "Please go in and ask. I am not the Boss!"

After a bit of haggling over the prices, the Committee said they'd decided to award me the contract. They asked me to stay back to "take possession" of a truck full of fabric the next day. I did a little tango in my head. This was my first big order. I called Meena from the hotel that evening to share our break-through. The next morning when I woke up, I thought the sun shone brighter. After completing the documentation process at the office, I came back with 'one truckload of fabric'. We continued their production for a good two years. We were making about 30000 pieces a month. Business was good. However, the government enterprise was not being managed properly. This trend is especially common in government-run textiles businesses in India where promising government projects have failed due to unprofessional or poor management. For instance, in this case, I saw that their retail stores were showcasing the ready-made shirts and the fabric (from which it was made) at the same counter. The natural tendency of the buyer will be to start calculating the price - whether it would cost him less if he were to buy the fabric and get it stitched rather than the readymade shirt made out of the same fabric. As a result, shirts were not moving.

Eventually, they landed up with a huge stock due to erroneous marketing policy or perhaps, the utter lack of one. Later they did manage to announce a 50% discount or *'Buy 1 Get 1'* scheme. But this too, failed. The shirts were not showcased well, they lay crumpled and looked shoddy, and the poorly presented goods failed to attract customers. Finally, they stopped giving fresh orders.

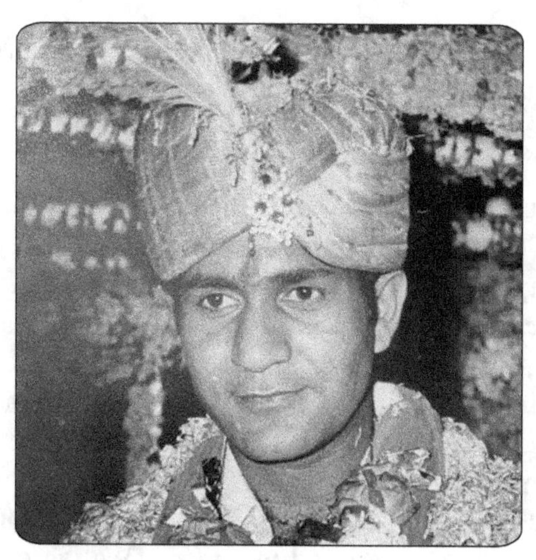

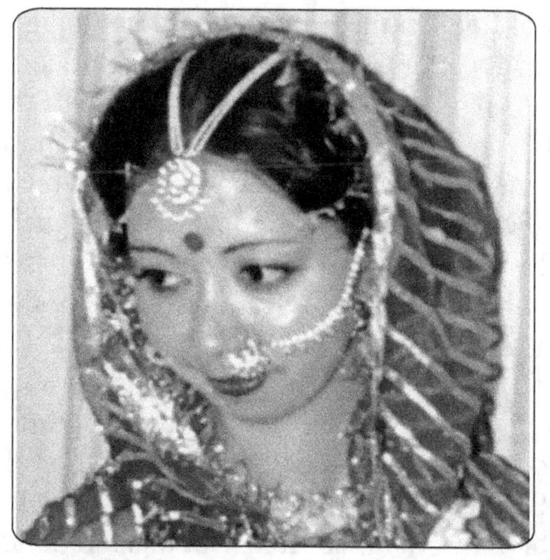

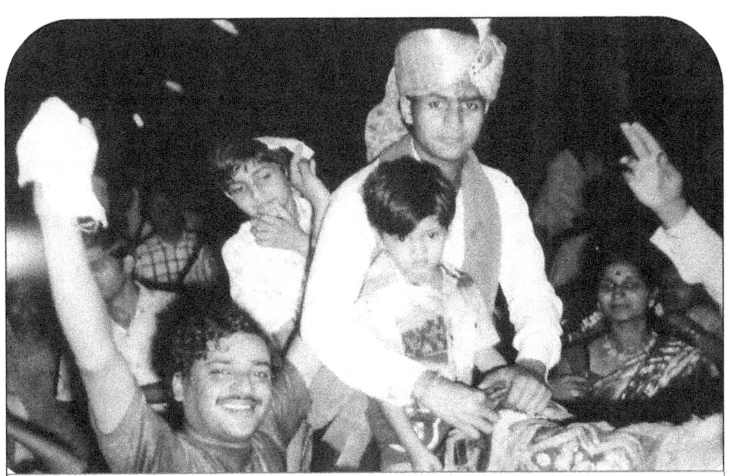

Exuberant Smile!
My friend Vinnie, in black round neck T-shirt, hands raised
jubilantly, by the side of the ghodi (horse)

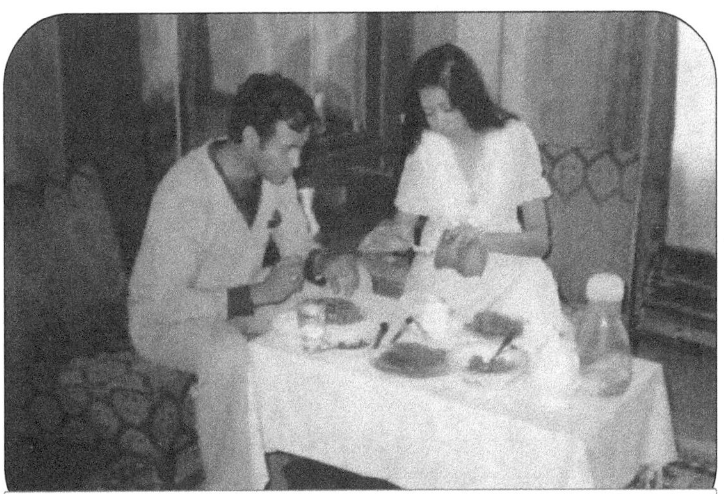

Stay at the Houseboat in
Dal Lake, Srinagar

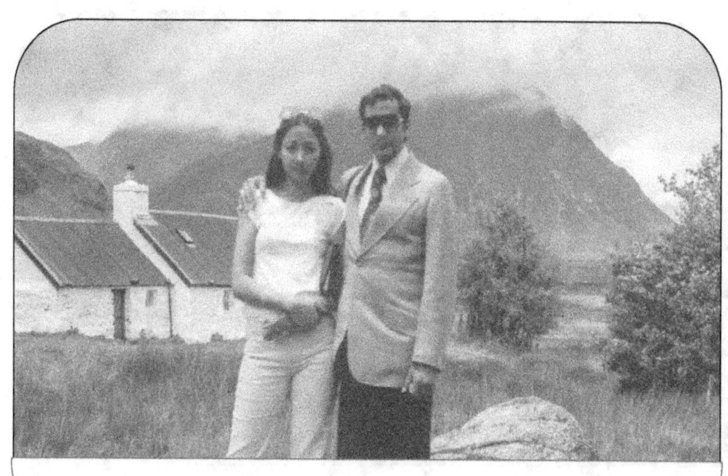

The Honeymoon. 1980.

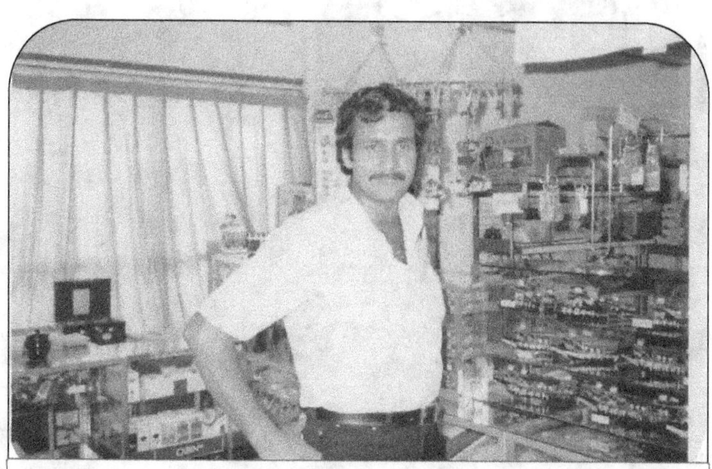

On his first overseas trip to Japan

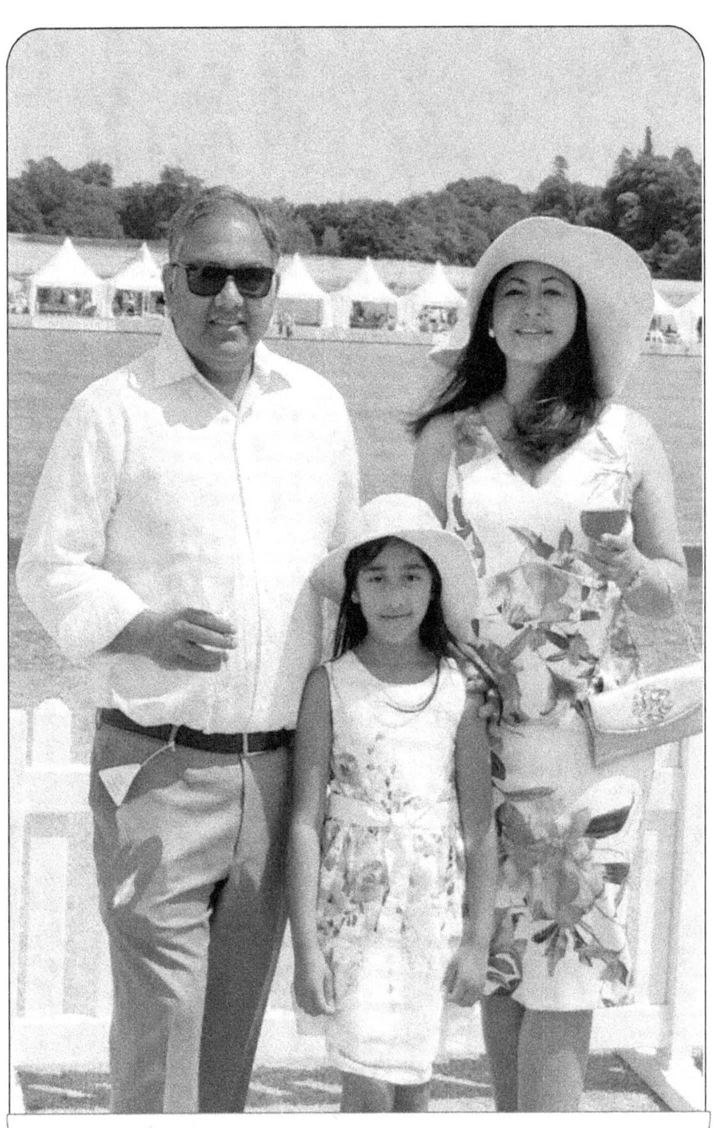

The Light of our Lives
Vikash, Shilpi and Zara

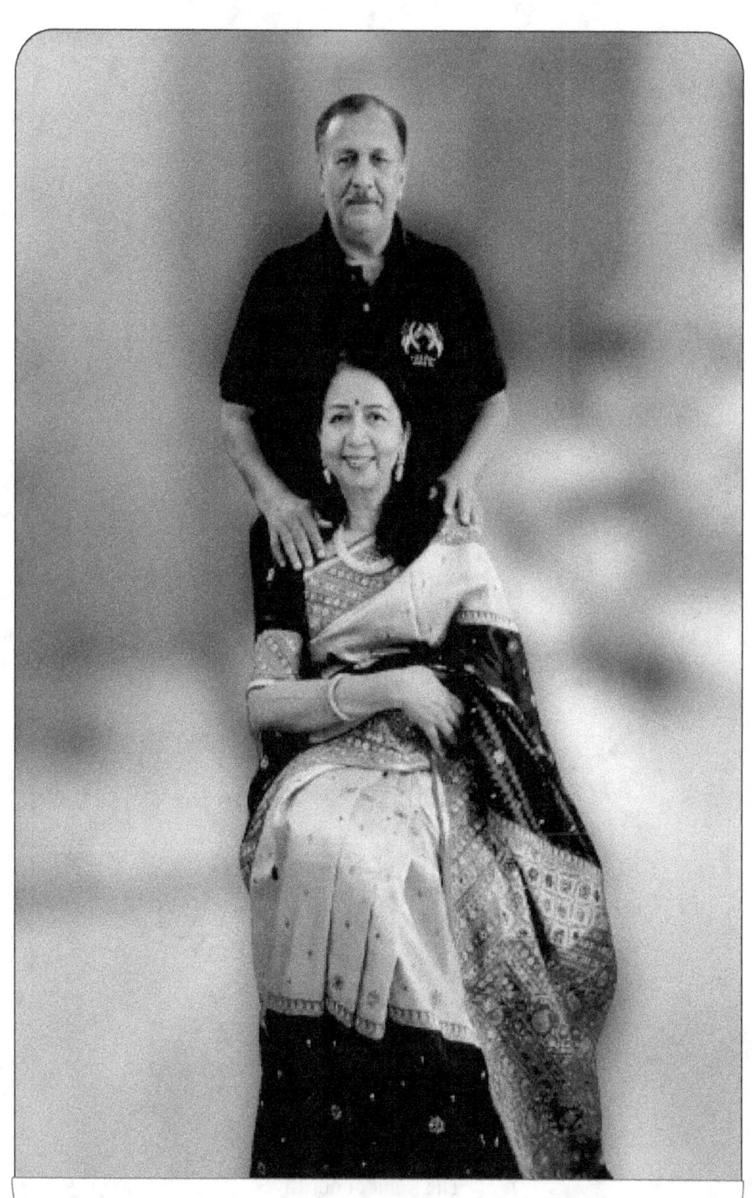

With Meena

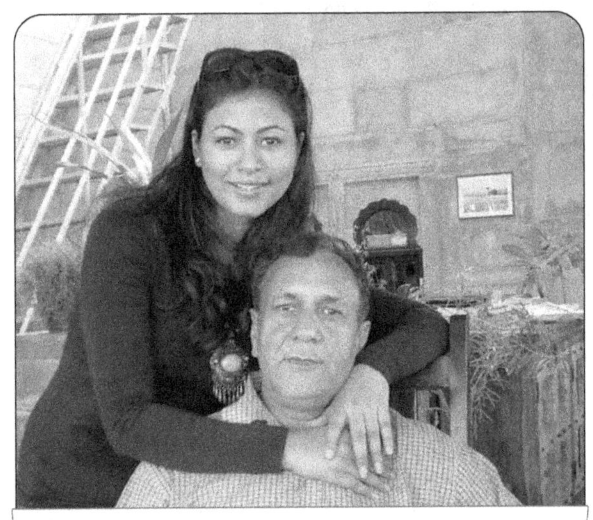

With Shilpi

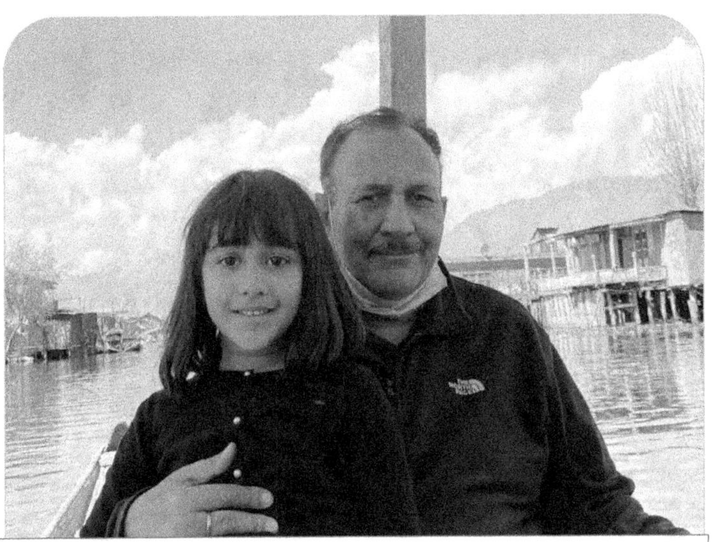

With Zara

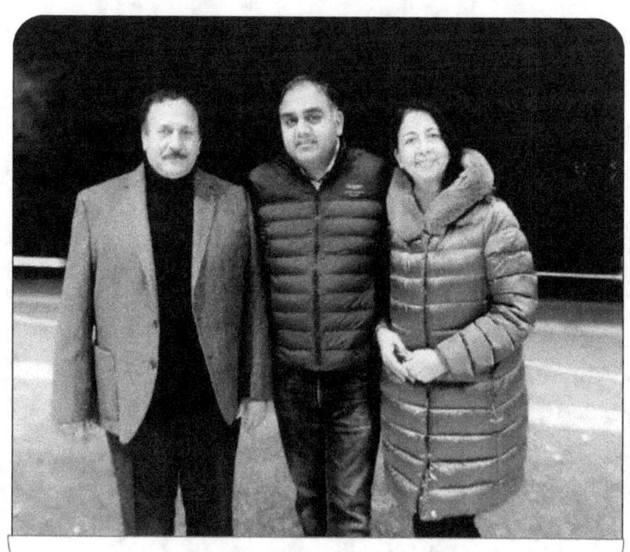

Arvind Aggarwal, Vikash, Meena

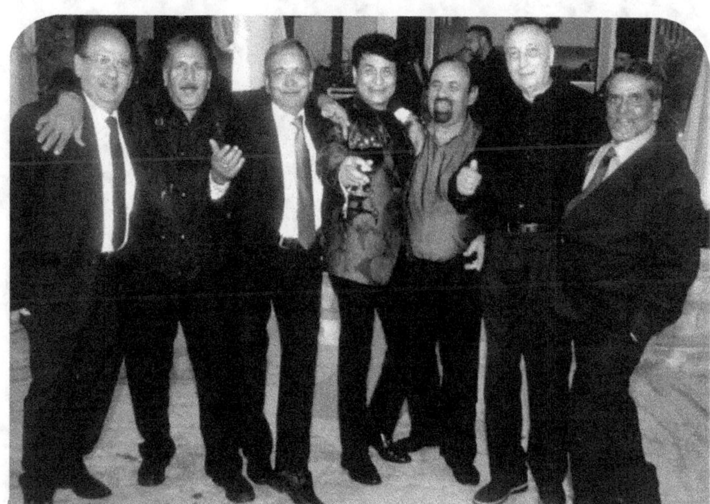

With MGM 70 Friends
Left to Right- Dr Rajesh Loomba,Dr Arvind Aggarwal,Dr K.K Singh,
Dr Rakesh Sahni,Dr Anil Saggar, Dr Ashok Bakaya, Dr Rahul Kondoliya

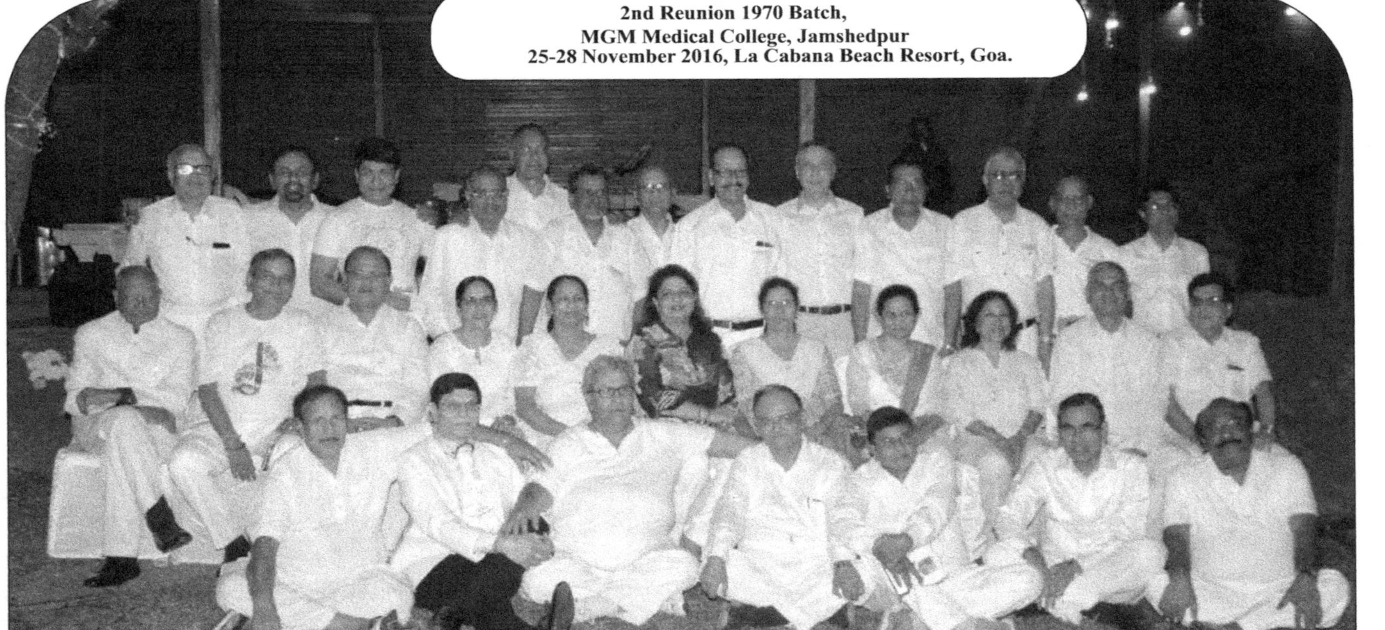

Left to right, Bottom row.

Dr Arvind Aggarwal,Dr. Ashwani Trehan,Dr. Pradeep Ganatra, Dr.Kishore Parekh,Dr.Vinod Kumar Singh,Dr.I.P.Mittal,Dr.Kiran Shah

(Middle row) Dr. Bharat Bhushan,Dr. K.K.Singh, Dr. B.K. Singh,Dr. Surinder Kaur,Dr. Reeta,Dr. Madhu Chopra,Dr. Charulata,
Dr. Srirekha Reddy,Dr. Sheeba Pillay,Dr. Ramprakash,Dr. Praveen

(Top row) Dr Ghanshyam Doshi,Dr. Anil Saggar,Dr. Rakesh Sahni,Dr. Naresh Gupta,Dr. Pramod Jaiswal,Dr. Rahul Kondoliya,
Dr..Satinder Singh, Dr. Ashok Mishra,Dr. Ashok Beckaya,DrShyam Kishore, Dr.Anand Mishra, Dr. Surjit Devgan, Dr Pranab Choudhary

By now, I had built sufficient resources to travel abroad for business.

Chapter 9

EUROPE AND THE REST
OF THE WORLD

But making the 'Break-through' in the export market was very difficult. I decided to start with Europe. I made my first visit in 1983.

For three months, I had been sending letters and telexes, without any response till it was time for me to go. Those days, there was no concept of *One Schengen Visa*. Entry to every new country required a separate visa. As I started applying for visa, strangely enough, every embassy would want to know if I had a valid US visa. So, I applied for the US visa first.

At the US Embassy visa interview, a perfectly coiffeured lady officer looked at me and said,

"How do you convince me that you will come back to your country, . . . not stay back in the US?"

I asked the Visa officer, "What makes you think I

shall stay back? Please give me one good reason."

Without waiting for her to respond, I continued,

"In India, I have people who help cook my food, clean my house. ...I don't wash my clothes, I don't have to wash the utensils or make my tea. I have people help do everything for me! In the US, things happen rather differently than at home. Why would I want to stay back?"

The Visa Officer looked satisfied with my candid response and with a marked change in her tone and manner, she said "Sir, could you please send someone to collect your passport at 4 pm".

The same evening at 4 pm, I had a a US visa. This really made getting other visa easy.

I travelled to Europe for the first time in 1983, working my way through most of the major West European countries. After landing in Frankfurt, I went to Dusseldorf, Hamburg, Copenhagen, Oslo, Stockholm and Helsinki. Then I went to Paris, Amsterdam, Belgium, Luxemburg, Switzerland, UK etc. I did not get any order anywhere, people mostly just wanted the free samples. I was carrying samples in two large bags weighing around 30 kg and a shoulder bag of 10 kg for potential buyers plus a briefcase that contained important documents. By the end of the sixth week, my hands had developed blisters and a blue mark ran across my shoulder where the bag's strap rested.

To avoid renting a hotel room, I now began to travel through the night by Euro-rail and work during the day with my bags stowed away in railway-station locker rooms. Going without proper meals for close to two months was beginning to take its toll on my body and spirit. And I was sore and weary of sleeping in railway station waiting-rooms and sleeping cars. But my situation was desperate. I couldn't return without business . . . I had not many options!

My sister-in-law Neena lived at Monchengladbach, a small town near Duesseldorf. I sometimes went over to spend the weekend at her place to save money, rest and get my laundry done, before heading out again.

I was nearing the fag end of my visa term when Meena called one day from India to inform me about a telex that came from H & M in response to my request telex (I had sent out tons of innumerable solicitations for appointment with potential customers before setting out for Europe, and mostly, received no responses).

Meena said that I had an appointment on Monday at 9 am at their office on 17 Jacob's Berg Gatan, Stockholm!

This was my chance. It was a Saturday when Meena had called. I put my bags in order and got ready to leave on Sunday by the 4 pm train that would bring me to Stockholm around 7 am on Monday. This meant that I had sufficient time to freshen up my body (and my soul!) before I walked in through the doors of the H & M Office, Stockholm.

This was my chance.

I met the designated lady, Ms. Gunilla Hulten. She went through my collection, her eyes carefully scrutinising the samples while her ears listened to me speak. Finally, she looked up and looking at me closely, asked about the 'very-conspicuous' blisters on my hands. I told her about my ceaseless travel across Europe with all the different garment samples. She asked me then if I'd managed to get a lot of orders since I had been through so many countries. She could have been testing me, so I decided to be utterly honest. I told her sadly I had not received any business. By the end of our meeting, Hulten offered me two orders:

1. Girl's Shirts: 6000 pieces @31 per piece and

2. Boy's Shirts: 5800 piece @ 29 per piece
My first ever international business deal. And my client was H&M. It was incredible! Not being able to entirely believe my ears, I asked her for the order sheets. She said she would send it to India, but I wanted them in hand. She responded,

"Can you wait till later in the evening?"

I thought, "No! My money is nearly finished. And I'm hungry, thirsty and very, very, very tired."

I said, "Yes."

Bang opposite the H & M office on Jacobs Gatan street, stood a quaint little coffee shop. Since it was almost freezing outside, I decided to go in and wait there. I had spare money for only one coffee. As I was ordering my coffee, I told the guy at the counter, "I have to pick up my order from H & M in the evening at 7 pm, can I please sit in your shop till then . . . but I only have money for a single coffee". He said the sweetest three words in the whole wide world, "Sure, you can!" I sat there and sipped my coffee. The hours were slow to progress. After some time, the counter guy came around and said, "Hi! I'm making a coffee for myself ... do you want one too . . .?". I said, "No, thanks!"

He perhaps felt my hesitation, so he quickly added, "Don't worry, this one is on me . . . ." I was genuinely touched by his warmth but couldn't bring myself to say a "Yes!" So, I refused him very politely.

A little before 5 pm, the counter guy was once again by my side. He put down a glass of warm water on the table in front of me. While I was drinking, he said, "It's about time you went inside the H & M office, because the office closes at 5 and after that, the Security won't let you in."

So, I got up and went across the road into the H & M office and began to wait in the Reception area. The coffee machine in the corner reminded me of the counter guy. The thought of him made me smile and warm. The H & M office was just a short walk from the coffee shop, but I was cold. After a while, I got up and poured myself a cup of coffee. And then another.

Exactly at 7 pm, Gunilla emerged through the doors, a thick brown folio in hand, and instructed the receptionist, "There will be an Indian guy coming at 7 pm. Please hand him this folio".

The receptionist, pointing at me, remarked, "There is a guy waiting here since long . . . hope he is not the one . . .". "Indeed, he is!" and she turned towards me with a "Hi! There you are…", and handed me the brown paper envelope with a smile.

Thus, I literally "bagged" my first international export order. It was like a dream. My goals suddenly seemed to be at an arm's distance. My eyes were brimming, so I hugged my overcoat tightly. As I walked out into the street and hailed a cab to the station, there was a spring in my step.

That night, as I boarded the train to Oslo, the roadmap in my head was clear.

* * *

The YELLOW PAGES!

Transformed overnight from a depressed person into a successful exporter, I was a happy man. Getting off the train the next morning, I went straight to the Indian High Commission office.

I could sense that I was sparkling with a new-found confidence. I wore my ombre-blue suit with a generous bout of cologne; feeling (and hopefully, looking the part!) every bit an International Exporter! The High Commission fixed two appointments for me in Oslo to meet potential buyers. The first appointment wasn't fruitful.

In the second, I met a 6 ft. tall gentleman. His name was Mr. Tormod Froyland and his voice was gruff. Cigar in hand, he started the conversation with,

"Who do you work for?"

With the H & M ordersheets in my hand, I said nonchalantly, "H & M".

He exclaimed, "Oh! I work for H & M too. Will you work for me?"

I responded, "Of course, *Yes!*"

So we got down to work on making orders. By 7 pm he'd written me 10 orders of 2000 pieces each, that is 20000 pieces. At Rs 55 a piece, it was an order of a whopping Rs 1100000!

Not bad. Not bad at all…I almost patted myself on the back and left for the station without looking back. I came to Frankfurt to take the home-bound flight. So, at the end of my very own first export promotion trip in 1983, I had orders worth Rs 16 lacs (equivalent to Rs. 1.6 crore today). This was the beginning of our export business. At long last, I had finally managed the 'Breakthrough'.

Soon my travels became more frequent, spanning most of West Europe. I could capture a fair share of the West European garment market in France, Italy, Belgium, Netherlands, Switzerland, Germany, Sweden, Norway Denmark, Spain and Hungary in East Europe.

Business expanded and grew and we added more products. And I started marketing offices in France (Paris), USA (New York) and Hungary (Budapest). In the Hungary office, I had a small team of three girls,

Ildiko Nagy, Melinda Benkutii and Vari Judit, and our driver Samuel. While Melinda managed the office; Ildiko, Judit and me were constantly in 'the field' meeting buyers.

My daily sales in Budapest was close to 100000 pieces of T-shirts daily @ USD 1 per piece. We'd travel by car to different buyer locations, throughout the day. While I was in the front seat next to our driver, both Ildiko and Judit would be making calls from the backseat. We travelled with a file which contained all the important contacts and their phone numbers. We used to call it the YELLOW PAGES!

We had two Nokia mobile handsets. In the early 90s, these were really heavy phones, weighing about 400 gms each. Both the girls were on the phone continuously, trying to generate a greater volume of sales. It was salary plus incentive per sale. Whenever we found a potential buyer willing to buy, we would turn around our car for the buyer's office. Oftentimes, we would reach the buyer's office and collect advance payment in cash for delivery the very next day. This we communicated to Melinda who would prepare and keep the papers ready for next day's delivery.

Every morning, as soon as the Hungarian Reserve Bank opened (at 7 am), an assistant from Szentex would deposit cash in the Reserve Bank in Forints (the Hungarian currency), from where the payment after conversion into US dollars, would be transferred to the Central European International Bank (CEIB) to Szentex account. The payment in USD would then be credited to our firm in India as remittance against exports from India by the CEIB.

On receipt of payment from the MHB, the CEIB would issue goods release letter to Szentex, against which goods were delivered to the buyers from

Budacont container depot.

Hungary had just broken out of the erstwhile Soviet Union and it did not have a well established banking system to support import and export transactions. So, we devised a rudimentary system for running our trade transactions by ourselves!

It worked well for us and in a period of five years from 1990 - 1994, we established ourselves as a well-known and major garment exporter from India. Business was excellent.

We had such a significant share of the T-shirts market that we were selling almost 100000 T-shirts per day every morning (and that, against advance payment!).

In fact, we used to 'open' the rate of T-shirts in Hungary.

One day, we received a call from a buyer who wanted 2 million pieces of T-shirts for the Swedish election campaign. The colour of the T-shirts was to be white with their political party's logo printed on the front (chest). I did not have a ready 2 million white T-shirts in our stock. Hence, I negotiated a deal with large Chinese importers from whom I sourced the T-shirts and a Chinese printer in Budapest who could print the logo. The goods were exported
by trucks from Budapest to Stockholm, successfully delivering 2 million pieces in about 2 weeks' time. (I think what helped us garner positive market goodwill was our quick response time and committed execution).

Besides, we had a stable presence in the French market through many smaller buyers. In Oslo, we had an agent called Odd Hallan but he was quite small, buying only one container (1 container size equalled 40000 pieces) a month in summers. Since Norway was a very small market, we decided to drop it over a period of time.

Our business relationship with H & M from 1983 till about 2000, was long and productive. We regularly exported to H & M from India , and sporadically from Nepal and Bangladesh. And once even from Hungary. We onboarded the largest factory called KDS Garment Industries Ltd. Chittagong in Bangladesh to manufacture for us.

My experience of visiting the factory floor at KDS Garment was nothing less than phenomenal. This factory was owned by Mr. Khalilul Rehman, who was also the Chairman of the Bangladesh Shipping Corporation as well as the National Bank of Bangladesh. In addition, he was also a very big importer of powder milk for Bangladesh from Austra lia and New Zealand.

KDS Garment Industries was a spectacularly well-organised factory. There were some 2000 machines distributed into 10 units, all under one roof. These 10 units were vertically organised to cater to the different stages of manufacture and production, esp. the Store, followed by the Cutting dept, Rolling dept, Stitching, Thread cutting, Pressing and Packing dept. The entire Production process was 'quantified' rigorously. For instance, I noticed that the production per hour was displayed for every person (operator) on the production board. A miss in the production target would lead to a pay cut, and should the default continue, the person might even lose the job. This was smart but also scary!

With money, you can achieve most things at most places. But in Bangladesh, money makes just about anything possible. Has anybody ever heard of air travel without a ticket and without a seat in the aeroplane? Here's a stunning experience. Chittagong airport does not have a ticket selling counter at least, it did not have one back then.

It so happened that I was required to come to Dhaka

from Chittagong expeditiously. Tickets were purchased from the city office. Given the sorry state of the Chittagong city roads and the abysmally slow traffic, it took me forever to reach the airport. By the time I reached the *Check-in* counter, I found the flight had already left and my ticket became a 'No-show'.

So, I asked the guy at the counter about the next flight which was due in around an hour's time, and if he could somehow get me a ticket on it as it was not possible to go to the city and return in time for the flight. In response, he seemed to look through me and then look at somebody in the distance. I turned around to follow his gaze and I saw an airport clerk. Before long, and much to my astonishment, the clerk was fast approaching us with a toothy grin. "*Dada* (elder brother), what's the problem . . . Can I help you?", the porter was now by my side.

As I looked askance, the counter guy gestured to me as if to say, '*He will help you*'

The porter continued,"There is a man at the *Check-in* counter for the next flight. Go and pay him 300 *taakas* (Bangladeshi currency)."

So,he will come to my rescue for a cost. Fair enough. I was satisfied.

I went up to this *Check-in* counter guy and, telling him my plight, managed to persuade him to arrange a boarding pass for the next flight. For the cost as mentioned, which I paid. But much to my surprise, once the passengers' boarding started, the *Check-in* counter guy seemed to not know me at all, deliberately avoiding my gaze. Passenger after passenger would come, show the ticket, get the boarding pass and go on to board the flight. Except for me.

I kept waiting, and waiting and waiting. Occasionally, I would try to talk or even attract his attention but the counter guy seemed determined to not know me. Finally, once the last passenger had taken the boarding pass and left, he quietly came around and picking up one random bag from the conveyor belt, began to rub off the cross-mark on it. Once done, he put down the bag on the side. He now handed me a boarding pass and before I could begin to comprehend what had just happened, I was whisked off into the flight.

The practice, at the time of *check-in,* was that the cross-mark in chalk on every piece of luggage denotes that it has been screened and cleared. He kept out this one bag after rubbing off the mark on it and announced the seat number.

The baggage 'hanky-panky' was incredibly shocking! Almost instantly, one man in an orange T-shirt came running down the flight to get his bag cleared. In absolute horror, he saw his bag lying by the side of the conveyor belt. And he began to look around frantically for the Custom Officer.

In my heart of hearts, I prayed for the unsuspecting man, hoping he would find a way out and reach where he needed to be.

Once inside the plane, there were more surprises. I found I was not alone - there were two more persons who were standing and without a seat. The air hostess whispered into my ear that since the others did not get a 'seat', I shall have to travel standing, too. When the seat belt sign was switched on, she asked me to go to the lavatory and sit in there. And once the seat belt signs were switched off, I came out and stood in the aisle. It was a short flight, just over half an hour, so it wasn't difficult.

But the experience was nothing like I've known before. Around the world.

Chapter 10

FIRST, SECOND, THIRD . . . STROKE

On the home front, my little girl Shilpi was all grown up and back home after finishing her MBA from Strathclyde University, Glasgow that summer. On 6th June 2006, Shilpi married Vikash (who had also just completed his MBA for Carnegie Melon University USA). I found Vikash to be genuinely friendly, perceptive and very dynamic.

Vikash's is a journey I am truly proud of. From starting work, through campus placement, with Booz Allen Hamilton in London to the Barclay's Bank, London to starting his own investment management company VAR (VAR - Vikash, Ashish & Rajat) together with his two closest pals, that handles transactions of a billion dollars to launching the MONUMENT BANK in London, Vikash is a powerhouse of grit and gumption.

Shilpi and Vikash live at Queen's Gate in central London with my most favourite person in the world and their daughter - Zara. Zara, an 8-years old little angel sings *(bhajans),* dances (various classical forms) and generally has all of us dancing to her many tunes!

* * *

Tragedy is the most potent when it strikes unannounced.

2011. We have a Community Centre with an adequate sports arena where I stay (DLF 2 K Block. Gurugram).

My senior neighbour was a regular at Badminton. And every morning exactly at 7 am, he would call to wake me up and we would go play.

One morning, at the Community Center, there were these two young men playing Badminton. So, the two of us joined in as a team against them. I played aggressively but it was a very hectic game. After a while, I could sense being flushed and perspiring profusely.

Taking a break, I walked to the water cooler just outside the Badminton court for a sip. Unluckily, there was no water in it. I remember feeling very thirsty, hot and sweaty. But I returned to the court to finish the game. As I started to play again, suddenly all was dark. I fainted and fell down.

My neighbour brought me home. Meena quickly made a full jug of fresh lime water for me, but I did not feel well.

My right arm and right leg felt especially weak and unsteady. I was not able to walk. Observing that all is not well with me, Meena suggested that we go to the hospital for a check-up. I don't usually like to go to hospitals but that day, I immediately agreed.

We were supposed to leave for London the next day to visit my daughter Shilpi and son-in-l aw Vikash. At 8 pm, Meena took me to Medanta Hospital for a check-up, but they admitted me in the Intensive Care Unit. The emergency MRI showed a clot that had gone to the brain . . .

They started me on Heparin Pump to dissolve the clot. Now, a very fine balance must be maintained on a Heparin dose. If a high dose is given, it leads to bleeding and if it is less than the adequate dosage, it will result in clotting. Hence, only an experienced neurologist who prescribed it or someone especially in-charge, should handle the dosage.

At Medanta, almost everyone was allowed to fiddle with the Heparin pump. The junior doctors who came on 'visit' would play with the knob, casually rotating it left then right - altering the dosage to less or more. In the next three days, I suffered another brain stroke.

I had gone to the hospital with hemiparesis of my right side . . . now I lost my speech.

A few days later, a third stroke! This time around, I lost my urine control.

With every passing day, my condition deteriorated further. Meena, now joined by our daughter Shilpi, was distraught. I'd suffered 3 strokes in the 12 days of my hospital stay. It was as if I was lying-in-wait for the final stroke to bid a final goodbye. Meena and Shilpi fought the hospital and got me discharged from Medanta. They shifted me to Sir Ganga Ram Hospital under the care of Dr. P K Sethi, a renowned neurologist.

Initially, we could not get a 'bed' in the ward, so we had to stay on a bed in the corridor. But my treatment had begun. And begun well.

Dr. Sethi 'fixed' the Heparin dose once and it

continued through the next few days.

At Medanta, we were told that I will never be able to travel, which I so loved. Besides, export business requires hectic travel. Although it caused me huge losses, I closed down the European offices and my factory to exit export business entirely. I was put on blood thinner which meant even a slight injury could cause uncontrollable bleeding and death. And life would never be normal again.

After 8 days of my stay at Sir Ganga Ram Hospital, I returned home, walking and on my feet. I felt almost recovered.

* * *

Hit "Refresh"

Doctors had asked me to quit smoking. A chain smoker (with a daily quota of 2 packs of Marlboro!) for the longest time, I gave up smoking in one go.

And so, I was BACK!

Given another shot at LIFE.

One of the first things I did was join 'Fitness First', a new gym in my neighbourhood. No matter what, I was religiously at the gym everyday from 6 am to 10 am.

Gymming included an hour of mixed exercises and a 45 minutes' yoga session, followed by 30 minutes of steam/sauna. The rest of the time was spent reading the newspaper, enjoying tea/coffee or juice and making lots of friends in there. Two years later, I was physically and mentally stronger than I was before the stroke. As on this date (as I write), I am absolutely well. I travel, I drive, I play sports, I do everything they told me not to do.

Once I recovered, I began to think of other business options for survival. A few years later, we built a few rooms on the first and second floor of our house to offer them on rent to girls and ladies looking for 'Paying Guest' accommodation. Surprisingly, the rooms were quickly taken and we realised how large is the urban job migration in Gurugram. The ladies were working in various multi-national organisations such as PWC, E&Y, KPMG, Deloitte, etc. Our accommodation rental business took off and began to thrive, allowing us a decent income. We even rented three more buildings and converted them into PG accommodations. So we had around 42 rooms across 4 buildings, with approximately 120 ladies working in professional capacities in different corporate entities. It would go full for most of the year. However, Covid struck early in 2019 and caused significant damage to our enterprise, with most ladies leaving for home due to the pandemic. We were compelled to surrender the additional buildings.

However, our own building continues to host ladies and girls looking for a home away from home.

Part V

Home Is Where Health Is

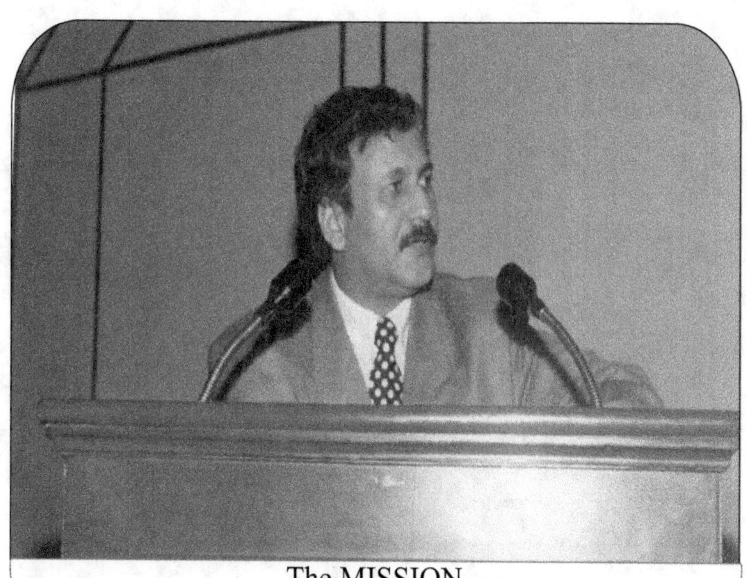

The MISSION
Explaining the Universal Healthcare Project to around 200
IT Companies at FICCI Auditorium, New Delhi (India).
1995

From: Bob Phillips <bphillip@online.no>
To: Dr. Aggarwal <technot@bol.net.in>
Sent: Tuesday, December 11, 2001 01:37
Subject: Re: NORWEIGIAN PARTICIPATION

Hi Doc,

I'll answer your questions as best I can, within the text of the message you sent me.
----- Original Message -----
From: Dr. Aggarwal
To: Bob Phillips
Sent: Saturday, December 08, 2001 7:26 AM
Subject: NORWEIGIAN PARTICIPATION

Dear Bob,

Shall be gratefull for the following tentative information

1.. Approx. value of finnacial support of TELENOR AS in Pilot Project
b.. Approx. value of finnacial support of TELENOR AS in Central Hub .
c.. Approx. value of finnacial support of TELENOR AS in Publicity for the 'Doctor's Training Course'
  *   Telenor is currently considering the above three activities as the total Pilot Project. I believe that they are working on a budget of NOK 8 to NOK 10 millions.
1.. Approx. value of investment of TELENOR AS in Seamless Services in the Joint Venture Entity with TTTCL
  *   Telenor's investment in the JV for setting up the seamless networking service will be considerable, most likely in 10's of millions NOK.
1.. Approx. value of Businesst expected by TELENOR AS from SMC Project
  *   I haven't been privy to their calculations. I believe that they have taken your figures as the basis, and have calculated out from 1000 SMC over five years.
1.. Approx. value of Business expected by TELENOR AS outside the SMC Project
  *   Again I haven't been privy to these calculations. Judging by my own thoughts, I would say that there is considerable potential in India. The level of system software sophistication and the very simple nature of the networking services available today, should provide tremendous growth in added value networking in India for the future. There is a lot of ground to be made up.
1.. Copies of MoUs, & JVs in other Countries for smilar kind of Projects
  *   I'm not sure whether this kind of information is available. To my knowledge they have had projects in United Emirates, Kuwait, Malaysia and Slovakia.
  I'll check if any of the MoUs or JV documentation is open to the public.
1.. Business Plan for India, Neighbouring Countries & Other Countries
  *   I'm sure Telenor will be generating a business plan as part of their process of establishing business in India. I would imagine that you will be involved in this process, particularly when gathering markets information about India, and clarifying regulative issues.
1.. MoU with Rikshospitalet
  *   Vinod and Dag will most likely be entering a contract with Telenor for their involvement in India

during the pilot phase. Later I would imagine the Rikshospital will enter into a contract with TTTCL for referrals, both from the SMCs and from Rikshospitalet to specialists in India.
1.. MoU with Mr. Robert Phillips
  *   I'm meeting with Håkon tomorrow to disuss t

Telex from Robert Phillips regarding Telenor's interest in our project

Chapter 11

THE VISION

The Vision :Emerging centrestage on the
Global Healthcare Map - India

I used to travel quite extensively for export marketing. After one such export marketing trip to Sweden in 1993, I was returning home to Delhi via Frankfurt. In the Frankfurt - Delhi flight, I was seated beside a gentleman who, by chance, had exhausted his supply of cigarettes. And I, of course, had enough on me! So, I offered him one. And that started the conversation.

His name was Deepak Srivastava. He was a Director of an IT Company and was travelling on business. It was now his turn to ask me my plans for life.

It was a simple enough question. Except that it set me thinking. I told him I wanted to 'do something' for the Healthcare industry. Deepak thought I was a busy exporter, avid traveller and accomplished businessman. Nonplussed, he asked me to explain. We started talking and the conversation lasted the next 8 hours till we touched down in Delhi.

Back to Delhi, Deepak and I met frequently over 'a cup of tea', discussing and debating how we can do 'It'. *The idea* began to take a rudimentary shape. Two years went by, yet we hadn't quite managed to make a break-through. We needed to build a delivery mechanism to translate the idea into reality. That's when we decided to invite diverse IT companies and present them with 'The Idea', and brainstorm together for a technological solution towards it s implementation.

The conference was attended by around 200 of the most prominent IT companies in India. *The Idea* generated great excitement and even promises of commitment, but not much of a tech solution. But every week, about 2-3 IT companies began to visit my office. I converted a small cabin in my office into a presentation room where I installed a TV and VCR. Here, visitors could watch an audio-visual simulation of the idea as I'd visualised it.

My **IDEA** was to develop a *Digital Medical Centre or a DMC* at the smallest and the remotest level, to realise the vision of **Bringing Quality Healthcare to the Last Person in the Last Village** .

A DMC with standardised digital medical equipment, 'manned' by junior physician(s) and backed by virtual consultants, can be set up just about anywhere, in both urban and rural areas but also in conflict-ridden zones or places that are adversely impacted by natural calamities. They can be installed even in trains and ships, as much as airports and rail stations.

Thus, there will be a network of state-of-the-art Digital Medical Centres spread across the country (to begin with), on the lines of the Mother Dairy milk booths in every corner, ensuring *last mile healthcare connectivity*

The Digital Medical Centres or DMCs shall be hosted on geographical spaces of no more than 200-300 square feet and will be run by an MBBS doctor(s) on franchisee basis. They can be set up just about anywhere and every DMC represents a digital hub or network that connects the common man/ woman/ child to a virtual global hub of consultant-specialists, physicians, hospitals and pharmacists.

Just like in a hospital OPD, the Doctor at the DMC will 'record' the pa tient history, only that now such history and complaints will be uploaded on an Electronic Medical Record (EMR), on a digital infrastructure powered by a **Universal Healthcare virtual ecology**.

The Doctor will then proceed to do a general examination on a high-defin ition General Examination Camera. The digital pictures will be uploaded and attached to the patient's file date-wise and item-wise, with minute details and colours. The lungs and heart examination will be done through a digital stethoscope. The heart's and lungs' sound will be recorded and put on the EMR. These can be replayed for accurate diagnosis and can be transmitted globally as an audio album like we transmit songs and music. The ECG will be done on the paperless digital ECG machine and similarly placed on the patient's EMR.

Examination of the skin, eyes, ears, nose and throat will be done through the digital dermoscope, ophthalmoscope and ENT-scope respectively - with all these functions being integrated into the multipurpose high-definition digital camera. The images and videos thus captured are of diagnostic quality and are placed in the EMR file.

A digital microscope shall be employed for the minute examination of blood and urine samples and the images on the slides shall be similarlyuploaded. In case required, a digital X-ray machine anddigital Ultrasound machine can be accessed at the DMC.Digital images from X-ray, Ultrasound, CT scan, MRI etc., can be uploaded and attached to the EMR together with the reports in the text format.

The patient file is now complete. The images, sounds and videos are of diagnostic quality (in a first-ever revolutionary innovation!).

In contrast to the present system where patient information is usually recorded by hand; here, the patient information is recorded accurately through voice, images, text and video format. This mode helps create a virtual patient (which is far better for accurate diagnosis) who can be transported globally, stored in the soft copy format and is retrievableanywhere globally irrespective of the geographical location of the patient or the physician.

The doctor viewing the file will prescribe the necessary treatment - this prescription shall now be attached to the patient file. A copywill be mailed to the chemist with patient ID and relevant details. The patient's EMR (inclusive of the video files, sound files, image data files and interactive video conference data) shall be available on Cloud for future reference.

In case where the patient needs consultation with a Specialist, the Doctor at the DMC shall connect with the desired Specialist. The patient's EMR will then be retrieved and shared with the Specialist Consultant. The Consultant can be located just about anywhere. Where such Consultant is remotely based, such Consultant can see and hear the patient, examine the medical history, investigations' results, even see (in real time!) the examination being done by the Doctor at the DMC or conduct the said examination himself/herself and advise the Doctor at the DMC on further course of action regarding investigation and treatment.

Like previously, the patient's EMR gets updated and stored in Cloud for subsequent references. Available as audio-visual-text file, this recorded history of the patient will be available to all Docto rs/Consultants in the future. It's a one-time record. In this way, a virtual patient and virtual consultant is created. And one can entirely bypass the complicated record-keeping by going without storing the various files for various ailments with different doctors and different hospitals. Indeed, the proposed system automates record-keeping and helps track and treat ailments for every patient, based on one holistic patient history across ailments and time frames of their occurrences.

The *round-the-clock* availability of Consultants is now real and can ensure zero wastage of time in treatment. DMCs also have multi-focal video-conferencing facility, especially effective in case of serious or critical patients where the physician/consultant can get opinions from other Specialists and/or institutions in India and abroad.

Thus, the patient can now, for the first time in the medical history of the world, directly access the best clinical expertise that there is. And this without having to suffer hefty expenses or the inconvenience of travelling or finding a helper/companion to help achieve all of this.

In case the patient requires tertiary care or surgery, he will be referred to the appropriate hospital.

So, this translates into benefits for all stakeholders.

For the PATIENT:
- The hospital comes home!
- Zero waiting time,
- Maintains social distancing,
- Cuts exposure to crowds and infections,
- Better and safer personal data storage,
- Digital EMR for data accuracy,
- Reduced malpractices and
- Reduced costs and inconvenience.

For PHYSICIANS ,
- Now there is a greater catchment area,
- Increased time at disposal and
- Fundamentally reduced overheads (such as car running and maintenance, c abin rent and overheads).

For GOVERNMENTS
- Generates self employment and
- Ensures quality healthcare for every citizen irrespective of geography.

* * *

Behind the Scenes

For a system that connects the last person to a global healthcare hub, we need a robust remote communication system.

Over 25 years ago, when I first encapsulated the idea and started to work towards bringing it to life, there was neither the ground nor the environment where it could germinate. For starters, there was not even the requisite bandwidth to host *live* and interactive video conferences across geographies, forget the new global wi-fi standards for instant connectivity and seamless communication that are available today.[1]

But I was a man on a mission. To make it work anyhow, I installed 3 ISDN lines in my office with 128 Kbps (Kilobits per second) bandwidth each, to give us a collective bandwidth of 384 Kbps (this was the minimum bandwidth required for conducting an interactive video conference).[2]

At the time, internet connectivity was very expensive and just installation of the three temporary ISDN lines cost me a bomb. Besides, there was no sponsor (or 'Angel Investor') so I had to manage all the expenses on my own.

To reach quality healthcare to every man, woman and child in this country; was a giant leap of faith.

In the year 2000, we organised the 'show' that was attended by AMD USA and Riks Hospital, Norway.

As the giant 70mm screen crackled to life, we could see Vimal's (the patient) eyes, ear,nose and throat being examined, live from USA. It was nothing like anything anyone had seen or heard before. The sound of Vimal's heart beating echoed through the massive auditorium, as the awestruck members of the audience gazed at Vimal (as if from just across the table!) while he was actually being examined real-time in the US. There was pin-drop silence. It was a surreal experience. An unprecedented idea that had transported the patient to the chair right in front of every member of the audience. *A spectacle that had the power to usher in a new era of universal healthcare for every person* .

This was followed by a demonstration of a live robotic surgery conducted by Riks Hospital from Norway on a patient in Switzerland.

The idea was starting to create a buzz. We were asked to repeat the virtual patient examination and surgery experience for another set of audience at Pragati Maidan (an events venue) in New Delhi.

It cost us a fortune to do such shows and the three temporary ISDN lines would often suffer interrupted transmission and maintenance issues. But the money saved from my export business and the thought of the remotest Himachali villager in my heart kept me going. Despite the hurdles, I was passionate to bring *the idea* to life towards ensuring healthcare to all and fundamentally transforming the healthcare landscape of my country.

We began conversations with different satellite companies who could rent us transponders or install VDAT on DMCS, but the cost was prohibitive and most importantly, the technology wasn't yet there.

We then discussed the proposition of saving data on servers. But servers could only save data in megabytes (Mbps), so a single server, at the most, could save only upto a few patient files.

This was the fag end of the 1900s when the first Pentium computer had just been launched in Dubai at a mind-boggling price of Rs 12,5000 and the like in most other low-income and middle-income countries. Of course, it was not available in India for a long time. The Pentium was a dream machine for most people and the IT industry was still in its nascent stages.

I had an internet connection (*mantraonline*) that took a fair amount of time to connect, I say 'fair' because at least, I knew that the connection would take time enough for me to grab a coffee or play with the dog in the meanwhile. Of course, it took hours to send an email with attachments, and attach ment failures were frequent, with several hours spent staring at the screen and praying for the connection speed to improve.

Today, most of us cannot imagine that past.

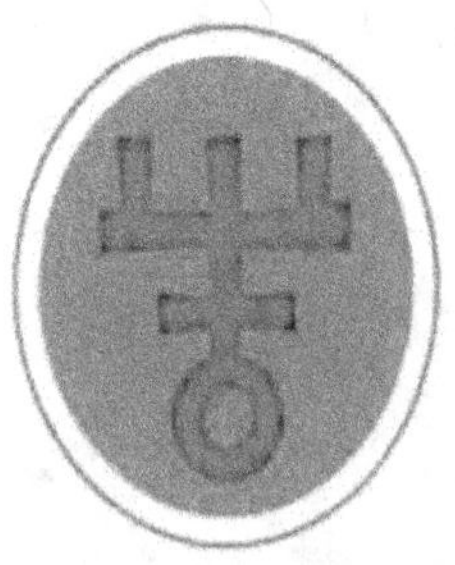

प्रगति मैदान, नई दिल्ली मे 14-27 नवम्बर 2001 तक आयोजित भारतीय अन्तरराष्ट्रीय व्यापार मेला 2001 के विशेष प्रदर्शन – नवीनतम प्रौद्योगिकी में उत्कृष्ट प्रदर्शन के लिए स्वर्ण पदक से पुरस्कृत

For Excellence in Technology Innovation at the
India International Trade Fair 2001
held at Pragati Maidan, New Delhi
November 14-27, 2001
Given this award of Gold Medal

विजेता **टेक्नो टेलीमेडिसिन एण्ड टेलीहेल्थ केयर लि.**

To **Techno Telemedicine & Telehealth Care Ltd.**

अध्यक्ष एवं प्रबंध निदेशक
इंडिया ट्रेड प्रमोशन ऑर्गेनाइजेशन
Chairman and Managing Director
India Trade Promotion Organisation

अध्यक्ष
निर्णायक मण्डल
Chairman of
Jury

Gold Medal Awarded for
Excellence in Technology Innovation in 2001

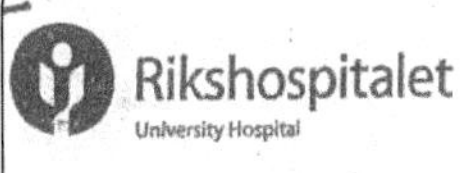

Rikshospitalet
University Hospital

The Deputy Director

Postal Address:
NO-0027 OSLO, Norway

Street Address:
Sognsvannsn. 20, Oslo

Switchboard: +47 23 07 00 00
Direct line: +47 23 07 09 81
Fax: +47 23 07 09 90

Reg. No. NO 970 897 771

Sevati Devi
Satellite Medical Centre Project,
India

Att: Dr. Aggarwal

Our ref: JK/01/01217
Date: 08.05.01

Letter of Intent

Rikshospitalet hereby confirms that it is our intention to participate in the planned Satellite Medical Centre project.

Our participation is dependent on agreement being reached regarding our precise role in the project, and on satisfactory financial arrangements being in place.

Concerning our role in the project, an indication of our current understanding is summarised in the attached document. The document describes how our contribution can complement that of the other Norwegian participants, and how it will fit within the scope of the project as a whole. The document does not constitute a formal offer, and should be regarded only as a starting point for further discussions. We remain flexible and open to new suggestions and proposals.

We propose that detailed discussion of financial arrangements should be postponed until our role has been clarified, and until a clearer picture of the financial arrangements in the project as a whole is in place.

We would also like to confirm that we will be delighted to take part, by video conference, in the function that is being arranged to mark the official start of the project. We will be in touch by email concerning detailed planning of that event.

Finally, we wish to express our gratitude and pleasure at having being invited to take part in your project, and look forward very much to our future co-operation.

Yours sincerely

Jomar Kuvås
Deputy Director

Letter of Intent by Rikshospitalet (University Hospital of Norway) to participate in Dr. Aggarwal's Project as Norwegian partner

Global Presentations

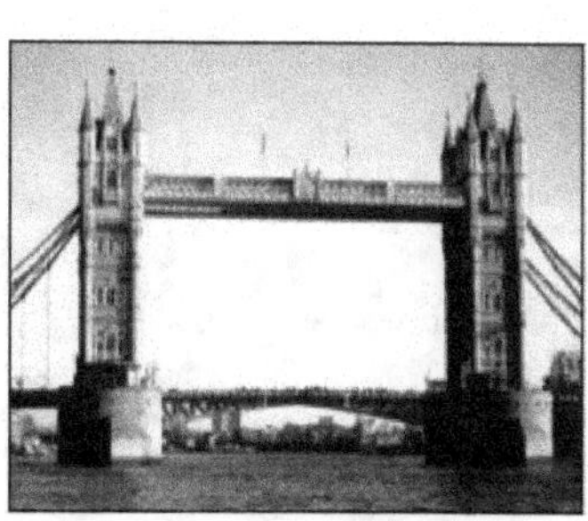

TM'99/113 presented in London at
Telemed '99 - a Conference of G8 countries
organised by
American Telemedicine Service Providers Association
*and Royal Society of Medicine, **London***

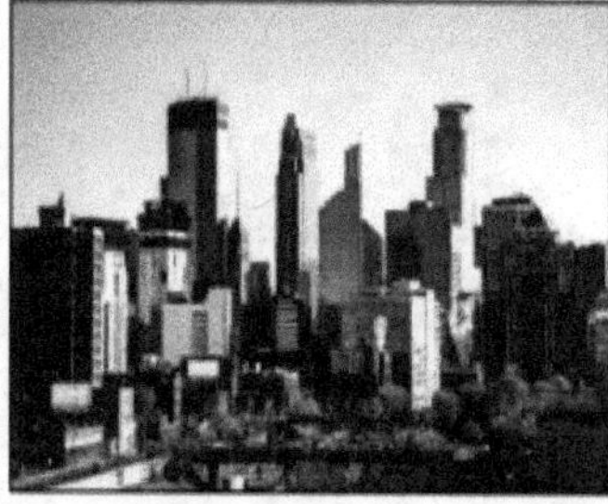

*Presented at **ATSP 2000 Conference** :*
Telemedicine & e-health : Common paths to the patient
*in **Minneapolis, Minnesota, USA***
in September 2000.

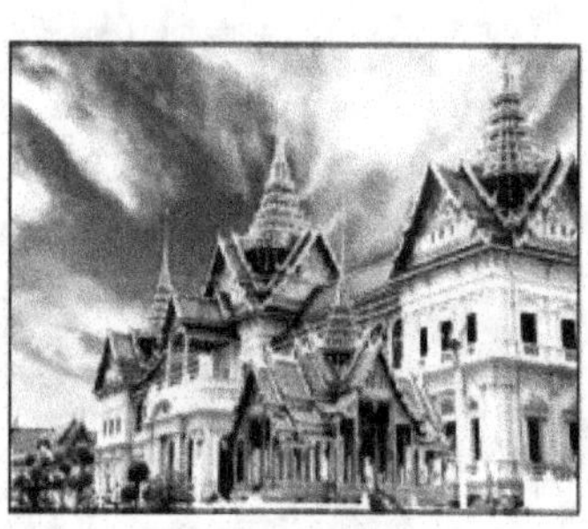

Sponsored by
United States Trade Development Agency
*to present at **Health care in Asia : New Technologies, -***
***New Options** - a competition of healthcare projects*
*from Asian countries in **Bangkok** in October 2001*

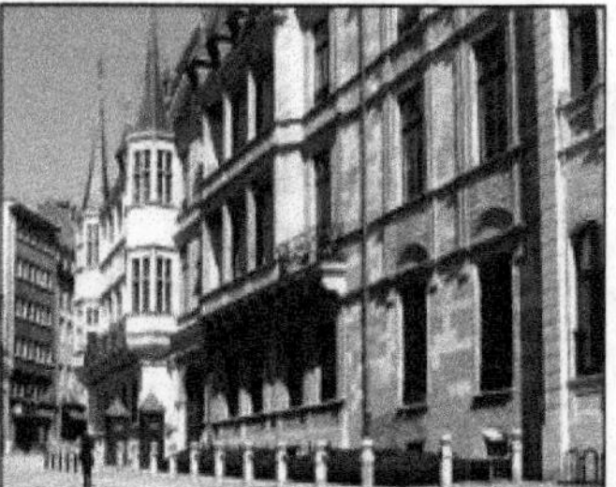

*Selected as a Key Project at **Telemedicine***
*and **Telecare International Tradefair, Luxembourg in 2002***
The Selection Committee had representatives from :
European Commission
Deloitte & Touche
Ministry of Health of G D of Luxembourg
Luxembourg Association of Medical Doctors and Dentists
International Telecommunication Union
Foires Internationales de Luxembourg

Dated: 4th December,2000

"Dear Dr. Aggarwal

I wanted to follow up with you on the potential of our involvement in the Telemedicine project. I would like to say that we are seriously interested in working with you. **We recognize the huge potential benefit from creating a project like this for the people of East Timor and for the doctors at our hospital, as well as the Yale medical and public health students who are working closely with GCHHR**

Please let me know what we can do to help, and how we can become involved in this project. I look forward to hearing from you.

Joanne Cossitt
Director
Griffin Center for Health & Human Rights

Letter of Interest and appreciation from Director
of Griffin Center for Health & Human Rights

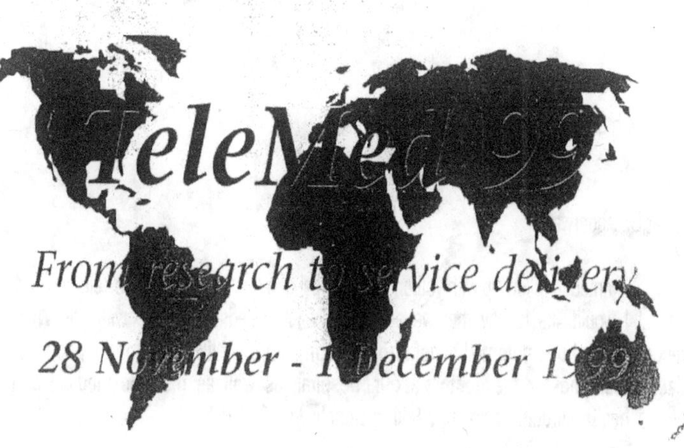

Conference Proceedings
Delegates' edition

Editors:
R Wootton
M Loane

TM99/113

Planning a low-unit-cost, high-volume satellite teleconsulting system

Arvind Aggarwal

Sevati Devi Memorial Hospital, Haryana, India

Correspondence: Dr Arvind Aggarwal, M-4/17A, DLF City, Phase-II, Gurgaon-122 002, Haryana, India (Fax: +91 124 364 699; Email: aggarwalarvind@mantraonline.com)

We have planned a low-unit-cost, high-volume national teleconsulting system. It envisages a central site manned by consultants from different specialties, with videoconferencing equipment, diagnostic equipment and appropriate peripherals. Satellite medical centres (SMCs) would be set up with videoconferencing links and diagnostic equipment, to provide patient examinations, investigations and consultations. To meet the traffic requirements of the network, a dedicated satellite with 10-13 transponders would provide broadcast- quality interactive videoconferencing at 2 Mbit/s per link.

The financial plan assumes that 15,000 SMCs would be set up in the private sector on a franchise basis, each costing Rs2,000,000-4,000,000 (Rs1 is $0.025, 0.026 euro). Another 5000 specialized SMCs would be set up in stages, attached to existing institutions and hospitals. Six doctors would be required to provide 24-hour cover in each SMC, and so the total requirement would be some 150,000 doctors. Each doctor would pay US$700 in instalments as a one-time life franchise.

At 2.5 patients/doctor/hour, 15,000 SMCs could service 657 million patient visits per year. If one patient visits an SMC five times per year, then this represents a service covering approximately 13% of the population of India. Doctors at an SMC would receive about Rs9500/month (almost what they receive in the government jobs at present). Consultants at the central site would receive Rs118,000/month. SMC franchisees would receive 22% profit after deducting all expenses. Each patient would pay a fixed charge of Rs50 per visit, which would include cost of examination, investigations and teleconsultation.

The contribution from the franchisees would cover the entire investment in the project. Since most of the expenses are fixed, profitability increases steeply as patient visits increase. At five patients doctor/hour, doctors' earnings would almost double. SMC owners would have a secure investment with regular lucrative income.

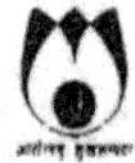

Director and the Faculty of
National Institute of Health & Family Welfare, New Delhi
cordially invite you to a presentation

on

Satellite Teleconsultation System in Health & Family Welfare

by

Dr. Arvind Aggarwal
Chairman & Managing Director

Sevati Devi Memorial Hospital & Satellite Medical Centres
at 3.30 p.m. on Friday, the 15th September, 2000 at NIHFW Auditorium

Shri A.R. Nanda
Secretary(FW), Government of India
has kindly agreed to preside

RSVP

610 0057 & 618 5696

Guests are requested to
be seated by 3.15 p.m.

(Map overleaf)

The presentation will conclude with a Question-Answer Session followed by Tea/Coffee

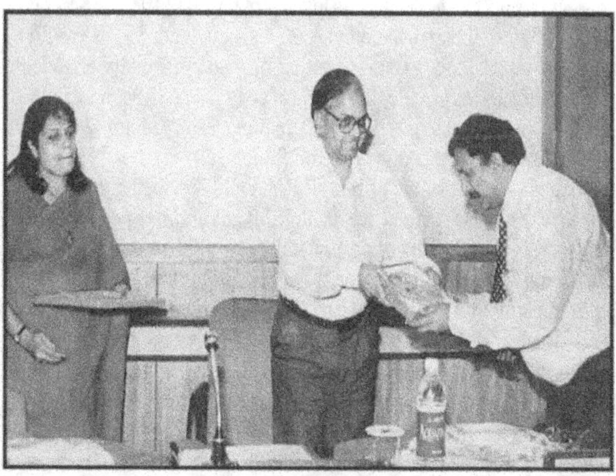

Shri. A.R. Nanda (Secretary, Family Welfare, Govt. of India) presenting a momento to
Dr. Arvind Aggarwal at a function held at the National Institute of Health & Family Welfare,
New Delhi on 15th Sept. 2000

Creating a Buzz!
Dr. Arvind Aggarwal being felicitated after a phenomenal
presentation and 'real-time' patient examination in 2000
when such things were unheard of

LARSEN & TOUBRO INFOTECH LIMITED

INFOTECH

Plot No. EL 200, Shil Mahape Road
TTC Electronic Zone, Navi Mumbai 400 701, India
Tel: 91-22-761 2571/75, 762 1100 Fax: 91-22-761 2580/82

Building relationships globally

Paranjape .S.T

9th August, 2001

Fax No: - 91-124-6364699

To
Dr. Arvind Aggarwal

This is to communicate to you that we are very serious and willing to join your consortium as major technology partners and also agree in principle to support the project technically and commercially.

Looking forward for long term fruitful association

Thanking You,

Yours Faithfully,

(Shripad Paranjape)
Senior Manager
Dotcom Startup Group – Navi Mumbai

Letter of Collaboration as Technical Partner.
Larsen and Toubro Infotech Company Limited,
9th August 2001

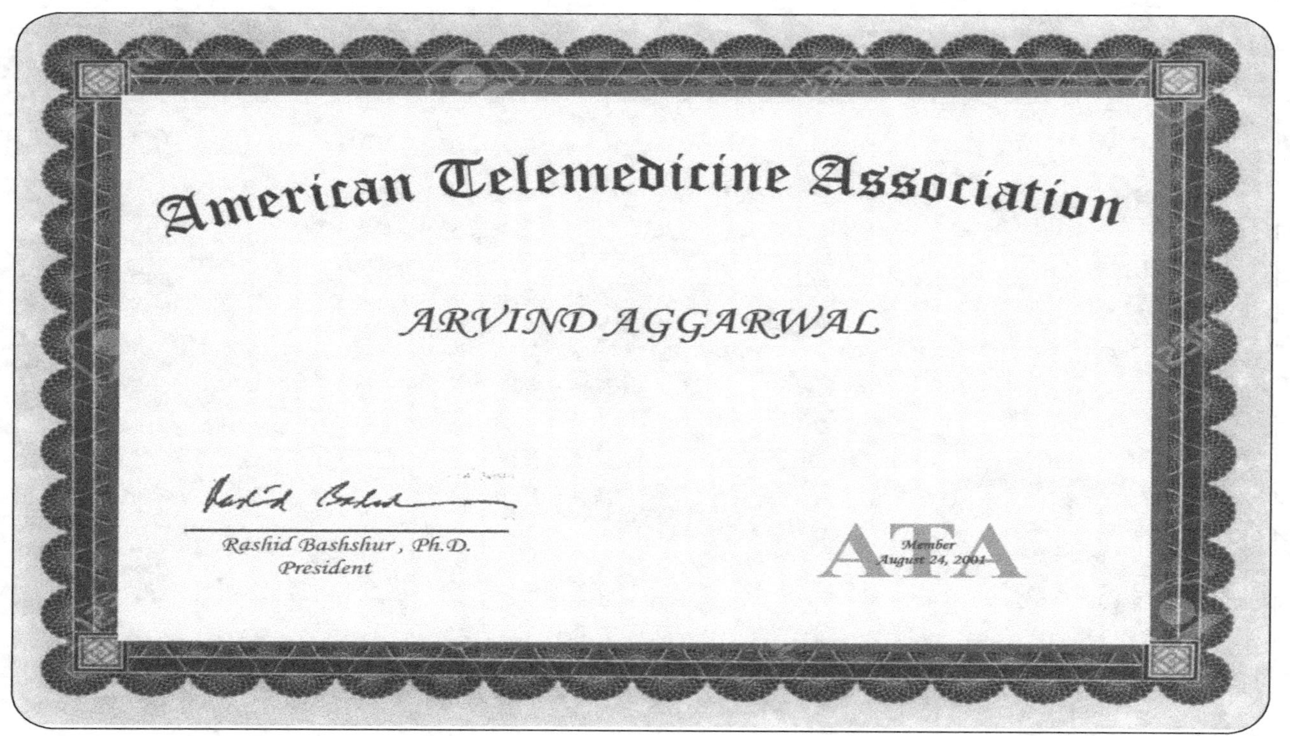

Certificate of participation in the conference held
by American Tele Medicine Association

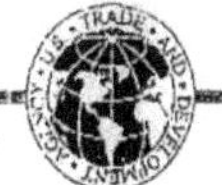

U.S. TRADE AND DEVELOPMENT AGENCY

September 21, 2001

Dr. Arvind Aggarwal, Chairman,
Technotelemedicine and Telehealthcare, Ltd.
M4/17A, DLF City, Phase II,
Gurgaon 122002
Haryana, India

Via Facsimile to: 91 124 636 4699

Dear Dr. Arvind:

On behalf of the United States Trade and Development Agency (TDA), I am pleased to invite you to participate as a project delegate in the **Healthcare in Asia: New Technologies, New Options Conference**, to be held in Bangkok, Thailand, October 17 - 19, 2001. The conference is being organized by TDA with the assistance of the U.S. Department of Commerce and 6 leading U.S. industry associations. The event will provide you with an unparalleled opportunity to establish or enhance relationships with some of the leading American healthcare information technology companies. In addition to yourself, other project delegates are being invited from China, Hong Kong, India, Indonesia, Malaysia, the Philippines, Singapore, South Korea, Thailand and Vietnam.

In sponsoring this conference, TDA recognizes the importance that new technologies will play in helping to develop new approaches to healthcare throughout the region. We also believe the exposure that this conference affords your projects will help hasten the timeframe for successful implementation. The conference program is designed to promote the productive exchange of project-specific information between you and the attending U.S. companies. At the conference you will present a brief overview of your project and meet one-on-one with leading U.S. companies interested in discussing your development plans and the specific needs of your project.

Moreover, you will have an opportunity to interact with fellow project delegates, representatives from various U.S. Government agencies, and leading officials from international financial institutions who could potentially assist the financing of your project. A U.S. Commercial Service Officer will accompany your delegation to the conference in Bangkok and help coordinate your program.

To confirm your participation as our guest, please fax your acceptance using the enclosed form to our contractor, MFM Group, Inc. (MFM), at +1.305.667.7840. Confirmation of your travel and logistical requirements will be sent to you separately by MFM once you have accepted this invitation.

We look forward to your positive response and to your participation in this exciting conference.

Sincerely,

Thelma J. Askey
Director

Enclosure: a/s

Letter of Invitation from
United States Trade and Development Agency (USTDA) to
participate as Project Delegate in the
International Conference in Bangkok -
'Healthcare in Asia: New Technologies, New Options

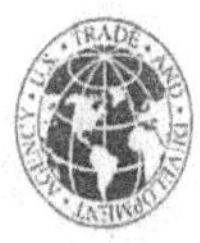

U.S. TRADE & DEVELOPMENT AGENCY

Health Care in Asia: New Technologies, New Options
A Health Care Information Technology Conference for South and Southeast Asia

Bangkok, Thailand • October 17-19, 2001

Project Resource Guide

Book I: Projects

Project Identification, Assessment and Characterization Conducted by:

Mark H. Spohr, MD
Medical Informatics, Inc.
PO Box 6984
Tahoe City, CA 96145
mspohr@nnk.com

under subcontract to:

MFM Group, Inc.
4856 SW 72 Avenue
Miami, FL 33155-5526
Tel: +1.305.667.4705
Fax: +1.305.667.7840
Email: info@mfmgroup.com
Web Site: www.mfmgroup.com

This report was funded by the U.S. Trade and Development Agency (TDA), an export promotion agency of the United States Government. The opinions, findings, conclusions, or recommendations expressed in this document are those of the author(s) and do not necessarily represent the official position or policies of TDA.

Mailing and Delivery Address: 1621 North Kent Street, Suite 200, Arlington, VA 22209 USA
Phone: +1-703-875-4357; Fax: +1-703-875-4009; Web Site: www.tda.gov; Email: info@tda.gov

Sevati Devi Memorial Digital Medical Centres Pvt Ltd
Project description by
United States Trade and Development Agency (USTDA) at
the 'Healthcare in Asia: New Technologies, New Options'
International Conference. pg. 1 of 2

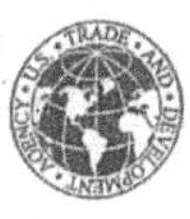 | **Technotelemedicine and Telecare, Ltd.** | 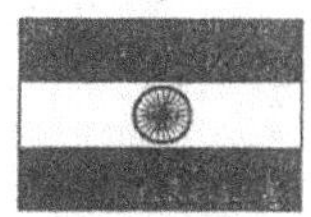

Project Summary: Clinic Information System, Telemedicine, EMR

Technotelemedicine and Telecare Ltd. has designed a dedicated telemedicine clinic that they plan to franchise and also contract with India state governments to build and run. Each clinic will have a complete full-time telemedicine link.

Project Description

Technotelemedicine and Telecare, Ltd. has designed a scalable telemedicine clinic that has the potential to be a very large project. They have designed a telemedicine clinic as a set system of 2,000 sq. ft. with six doctors, six nurses, and six technicians. They have designed a complete digital capture system that will use exam cameras, image capture, scanners, computer medical history, EMR to capture a complete medical encounter.

They plan to be able to ship the complete electronic encounter off a central expert consultant hub where the medical visit will be reviewed to maintain quality. This real-time consultation will require dedicated high-speed data links.

They are taking two approaches to funding the clinics. They have made proposals to 19 States to fund pilot projects (total of 250 clinics) that will be subsidized by the clinics. They are also planning a franchise arrangement with a franchise fee of Rs.30,000 (U.S.$ 666) and an initial investment of Rs. 45 Lakhs (U.S.$100,000).

The clinics include tele-consultation, with doctors at the Satellite Medical Centers interacting with patients and will have connectivity to the Central Hub with online transmission of voices and images.

Sponsor

The project is sponsored by Techno-telemedicine and Tele-health care, Ltd., which is a start-up company formed to design and implement this innovative telemedicine system.

Commercial Rationale

There is a large demand for private health care services in India.

This project will offer affordable health care with high quality due to the innovative IT design.

Sevati Devi Memorial Digital Medical Centres Pvt Ltd
Project description by
United States Trade and Development Agency (USTDA) at
the 'Healthcare in Asia: New Technologies, New Options'
International Conference. pg. 2 of 2

कोंकण रेलवे कॉर्पोरेशन लिमिटेड
KONKAN RAILWAY CORPORATION LTD.
(भारत सरकार का उपक्रम / A GOVERNMENT OF INDIA UNDERTAKING)
बेलापुर भवन, सेक्टर 11, पोस्ट बॉक्स नं. 9, सी.बी.डी.-बेलापुर, नवी मुंबई 400 614.
BELAPUR BHAVAN, SECTOR 11, P.O. BOX NO. 9, C.B.D. BELAPUR, NAVI MUMBAI - 400 614.

WE CARE

TEL. : 91 - 022 - 757 2015 - 18
FAX : 91 - 022 - 757 2420
Email: general@konkanrailway.com

No.KR/CO/MED/F-94/01.   Dt.10th October, 01.

Dr. Arvind Aggarwal,
Chairman & MD,
Technotelemedicine & Telehealthcare Ltd.,
M4/17A, DLF City,
Phase II, Gurgaon – 122 002
HARYANA.

        Sub: Telemedicine – Konkan Railway Corporation Ltd.
                . . . . .

        Kindly refer to the discussions dated 09.10.01.

        It is agreed in principle to have a pilot project for
one Telemedicine kiosk at Madgaon in the state of Goa and
Specialist hub at Belapur, Navi Mumbai.

        You are requested to kindly send a confirmed offer for
the same so that necessary required action can follow.

                                (Dr. V R Vatsai)
                                Chief Medical Officer.

The MOU which couldn't be implemented. . .
Memorandum of Understanding with Konkan Railways
towards developing mobile-DMCs

Dr. Nirmal Jain
Managing Director

January 18, 2002

Dr. Arvind Aggarwal
Director
Techno-Telemedicine &   <u>Fax No.0124-6389215</u>
Telehealthcare Ltd.
M-4/17A
DLF-II
Gurgaon – 122 002, Haryana
India.

Dear Dr. Aggarwal,

Sub : Telemedicine & Telehealthcare Project

With reference to above subject, as you are aware, we had number of meetings / discussions to understand the techno-commercial aspects of the project.

Prima-facie it appears to be a good concept particularly the objective of providing best health-care to common man at affordable cost by extensive use of IT and telecommunication.

In principle, we would like to support the project and would like to participate as an IT partner. Once we both work out details of various requirements, we could get into mutually beneficial arrangements.

Yours sincerely,

NIRMAL JAIN

Letter of Collaboration as Technical Partner.
Tata Infotech Limited,
18th January 2002

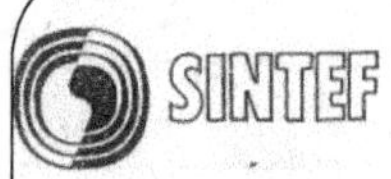

SINTEF Telecom and
Informatics

Address:
N-7465 Trondheim,
NORWAY
Location Trondheim:
S.P. Andersens v 15
Location Oslo:
Forskningsveien 1
Telephone:
+47 73 59 30 00
Fax:
+47 73 59 43 02

Enterprise No.:
NO 948 007 029 MVA

Dr. Arvind Aggarwal
Techno Telemedicine & Telehealthcare Ltd
India

Your ref.:	Our ref.:	Direct line:	Trondheim
	409520/JG7eh	+4773597085	2001-05-16
	40-UB012705		

Satellite Medical Centre Project, India: Letter of Intent

SINTEF Telecom and Informatics hereby confirms that it is our intention to participate in the planned Satellite Medical Centre project.

Our participation is dependent on agreement being reached regarding our precise role in the project, and on satisfactory financial arrangements being in place.

Concerning our role in the project, an indication of our current understanding is summarised in the attached document. The document describes how our contribution can complement that of the other participants, and how it will fit within the scope of the project as a whole. The document does not constitute a formal offer, and should be regarded only as a starting point for further discussions: we remain flexible and open to new suggestions and proposals.

We propose that detailed discussion of financial arrangements should be postponed until our technical role has been clarified, and until a clearer picture of the financial arrangements in the project as a whole is in place.

We would also like to confirm that we will be delighted to take part, by video conference, in the function that is being arranged to mark the official start of the project. We will be in touch concerning detailed planning of that event.

Finally, we wish to express our gratitude and pleasure at having being invited to take part in your project, and look forward very much to our future co-operation.

Yours sincerely
SINTEF Telecom and Informatics

Åge J. Thunem
Research Director

Encl. "Satellite Medical Centre Project, India: Project Management Consortium"

Letter of Intent by SINTEF Telecom and Informatics, Oslo for
participation in Dr. Aggarwal's Project.

SRI RAMACHANDRA MEDICAL COLLEGE AND RESEARCH INSTITUTE

(DEEMED UNIVERSITY)

1, RAMACHANDRA NAGAR, PORUR, CHENNAI - 600 116.

Prof. Sunil Shroff

M.S., FRCS (UK) D. Urol (Lond)

Head of Dept. Urology & Renal Transplantation Surgery

℗ Off : 4768403 Ext. 530
Fax : 091 - 44 - 4767008
091 - 44 - 6263477
Email : sshroff@vsnl.com

October 24, 2001

Mr Arvind Agarwal, M.D

Chairman

Technotelmedicine and Telehealthcare Ltd

Sevati Devi Memorial Ahospital

4/17A DLF City, Phase II

Gurgaon

Haryana 122 002

Dear Dr Agarwal,

It was a pleasure to have met you and interacted with you at Bangkok during the Asia Tele Health Care Conference

I am amazed that you have done so much to push the cause of Tele Medicine in our country and I must applaud you for your efforts. I wish you success in your ventures and I am sure with your efforts will soon be able to achieve the highest honours in what you have started

I wish to invite you to join the Medical Computer Society of India as a member and also to perhaps attend the National Conferenc to be held in March next year in Chennai. We shall keep you informed about the exact date nearer that time

Thanking you,

Yours faithfully,

DR SUNIL SHROFF

PROF OF UROLOGY & RENAL TRANSPLANTATION

Letter of Commendation from
Sri Ramachandra Medical College and Research Institute,
October 24, 2001

aggarwal

From:	Malina Jordanova <mjordan@argo.bas.bg>
To:	Dr. Aggarwal <_technot@bol.net.in>
Cc:	Dr. Arvind Aggarwal <aggarwalarvind@mantraonline.com>; Dr. Aggarwal <technot@bol.net.in>
Sent:	Monday, February 11, 2002 17:55
Subject:	Telemedicine & Telecare International Trade Fair - Educational Program

Dear Dr. Aggrawal,

We confirm the receipt of your contribution entitled:

World Class Health Care at Affordable Cost for Everyone - Everywhere

and its acceptance by the Selection Committee for presentation in the Educational Program of the Telemedicine & Telecare International Trade Fair, Luxembourg, G.D. of Luxembourg, April 10-12, 2002.

The Selection Committee was constituted of representatives from:

- European Commission - IST Program - Systems and Services for the Citizens - Applications Relating to Health;

- Deloitte & Touche, Management Solutions - Health Center of Excellence;

- Ministry of Health of G.D. of Luxembourg;

- Luxembourg Association of Medical Doctors and Dentists;

- International Telecommunication Union (ITU);

- Foires Internationales de Luxembourg;

which convened in Luxembourg on January 31st, 2002.

Your abstract will be included in the Abstract Publication, which will be part of Telemedicine & Telecare International Trade Fair Directory. It also will be loaded on the Trade Fair's website from the day of the presentation. Meanwhile the list of titles and names of the speakers will be added to the website in the next few days and will also be published in our e-mail newsletters. We'll inform you about the final schedule of your presentation soon.

Please be so kind as to inform your co-authors.

Acceptance of your contribution carries with it the OBLIGATION for you to actually present it at the Telemedicine & Telecare International Trade Fair 2002. If you or your co-author(s) feel that you may not be able to meet this obligation, you must give us IMMEDIATE notice, or no later than February 15th, 2002.

Letter of Acceptance of Paper Abstract and
Invitation for Presentation at
Tele-Medicine and Tele-Care International Trade Fair, LUXEMBOURG
February 11, 2002. pg. 1 of 2

Speakers also have to register as visitors to the Telemedicine & Telecare International Trade Fair 2002. Therefore, please send back immediately the visitors registration form (www.telemedicine.lu/eng/chap04/0402.html). If visa for travel to Luxembourg is required, please refer to the corresponding sections on the website (www.telemedicine.lu/eng/chap04/0404.html).

The organizers of the Telemedicine & Telecare International Trade Fair 2002 have also negotiated special hotel rates through the Luxembourg Convention Bureau. For more information and to make reservations, please consult our website at www.telemedicine.lu/eng/chap05/0502.html.

Carlson Wagonlit Travel is our official travel agency. Please contact their office in Luxembourg to find out about special travel discounts and to make the necessary reservations for your trip to Luxembourg (for Carlson Wagonlit contact details, see www.telemedicine.lu/eng/chap05/c0503.html).

Yours sincerely,

Malina Jordanova

Educational Program Coordinator

Telemedicine & Telecare International Trade Fair

****
Malina Jordanova, M.D., Ph. D.
Institute of Psychology
Bulgarian Academy of Sciences
Acad. G. Bonchev St. Block 6
1113 Sofia, Bulgaria
Tel: +359 2 979 32 04
E-mail: Mjordan@bas.bg

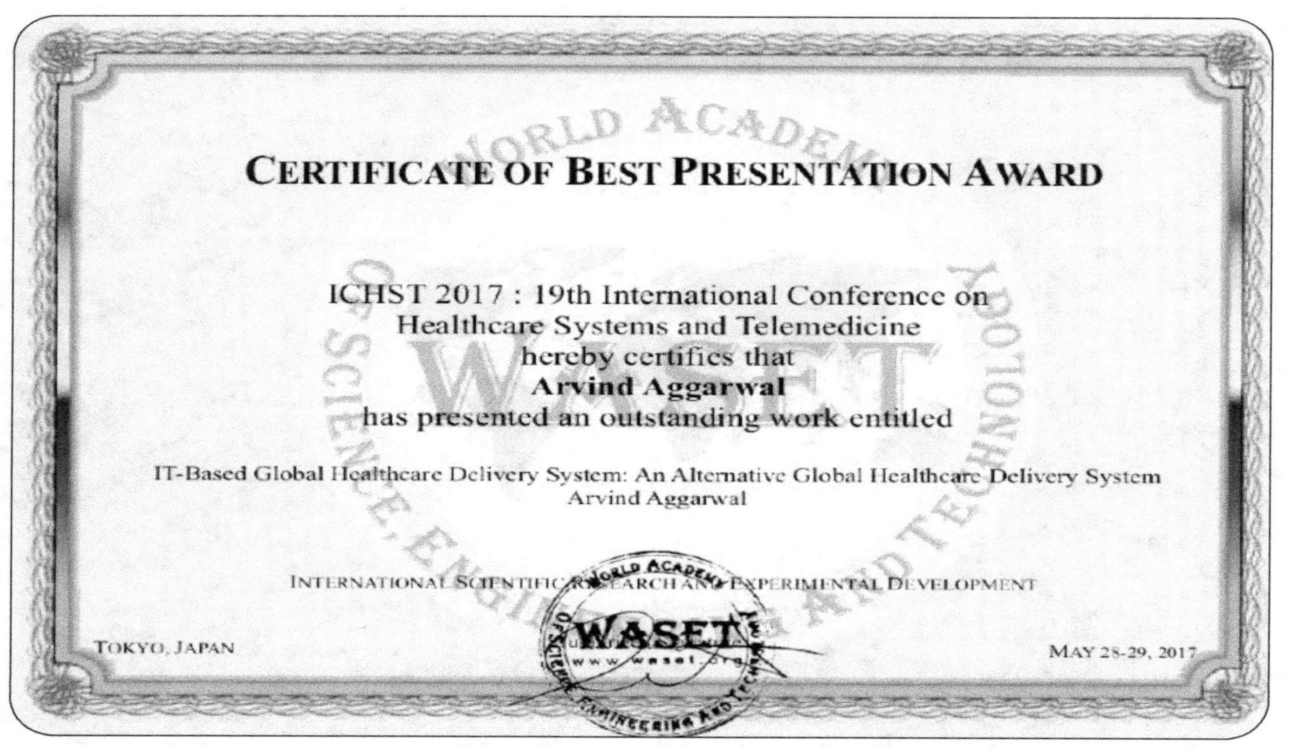

Numero Uno!
Dr. Aggarwal awarded the
"Best Presentation Award for Outstanding Work" by the
World Academy of Science Engineering and Technology,
Japan (2017)

From: <vinayakr@vsnl.net>
To: <technot@bol.net.in>
Sent: Monday, December 10, 2001 11:26

Hi Dr Aggarwal,

Pleasure hearing from you after long. I was wondering whatever really happened.

It is good to know the encouraging things happening at your end and with the project. When is the first commercial launch of SMC with konkan planned?

We are close to the launch of the ineractive portal for Escorts Heart and should be beginning web operations by early January. Also, a full-fledged implementation of a web-based HIS in an ASP mode is beginning January and we are currently in the process of finalising the agreements.

As I did mention to you during our Bangkok trip, it should be a pleasure being associated with your project, if possible in some hybrid way.

Here's wishing you all the best and would request if we could stay in touch.

Kind regards,

Ravi Vinayak

Letter of Commendation & Expression of Interest to be
associated with the Project from
Escorts Heart Institute
December 10, 2001

भारत को सचमुच जरूरत है टेलीमेडीसिन की : डॉ. अरविन्द अग्रवाल

अमेरिकी टेलीमेडीसिन सर्विस प्रोवाइडर्स एसोसिएशन की ओर से लंदन में आयोजित टेलीमेड-99 सम्मेलन में पिछले साल सेवती देवी मेमोरियल हॉस्पिटल एंड सीटी लाइट मेडीकल सेंटर के डा. अरविन्द अग्रवाल ने टेलीमेडीसिन पर बहुत प्रभावशाली प्रस्तुति दी। फिलहाल वे भारत में निजी क्षेत्र में एक पायलट टेलीमेडीसिन सेवा परियोजना पर काम कर रहे हैं। 'विज्ञान प्रगति' से एक विशेष बातचीत में उन्होंने टेलीमेडीसिन की बारीकियों, भारत में उसकी जरूरत तथा इसमें जुड़ी चुनौतियों के बारे में अनेक रोचक जानकारियां दीं। प्रस्तुत है बातचीत के महत्वपूर्ण अंश :

प्रश्न : डाक्टर साहब, सबसे पहले यह बताइए कि टेलीमेडीसिन वास्तव में क्या चीज है?

उत्तर : टेलीमेडीसिन मूलतः स्वास्थ्य सेवा प्रदान करने की वह प्रणाली है जिसमें डाक्टर दूर स्थित मरीजों की टेलीकम्युनिकेशन एवं इन्फॉर्मेशन टेक्नोलॉजी की मदद से जांच करता है, रोग का निदान करता है तथा इलाज करता है। इस प्रणाली में मरीज और डाक्टर एक दूसरे को देख सकते हैं, बातचीत कर सकते हैं। एक दूसरे से कुछ भी पूछ सकते हैं। ई.सी.जी., एक्स-रे, कैट स्कैन, एम.आर. आई. आदि की इमेज (तस्वीरें) कंप्यूटर विडियो फाइल खोलकर जांच सकते हैं। हजारों किलोमीटर दूर से ही डाक्टर डिजिटल कैमरों से शरीर के अंदरूनी भाग जैसे मुंह, नाक, कान, आंख, आमाशय, स्त्री-जननांग आदि के अंदर तक की जांच कर लेते हैं। हृदय की धड़कनें भी डिजिटल स्टेथस्कोप से सुन सकते हैं। यह मानिए कि जो काम मरीज के सामने बैठा डाक्टर कर सकता है, वह सब दूरसंचार टेक्नोलॉजी से डाक्टर दूर बैठे भी कर सकता है।

प्रश्न : क्या भारत जैसे गरीब देश में टेलीमेडीसिन जैसी चीज सफल हो सकती है?

उत्तर : भारत जैसे देशों में इसकी खासी उपयोगिता है। खुद हम जो टेलीमेडीसिन परियोजना शुरू करने जा रहे हैं, उसमें मरीज को सिर्फ 50 रुपये व्यय करने होंगे और इस राशि में वह एक्स-रे, रक्त, पेशाब, मल की जांच, ई.सी.जी. आदि करा सकेगा तथा साथ ही विशेषज्ञ डाक्टर की राय भी पा सकेगा। इतनी सस्ती जांच, निदान और प्रेस्क्रिप्शन क्या मौजूद परंपरागत प्रणाली में संभव है? नहीं, मौजूदा प्रणाली में इस सब पर करीब पांच सौ रुपये खर्च हो जाएंगे। ग्रामीण इलाकों में तो इस सबके लिए कई जगह जाना पड़ जाएगा।

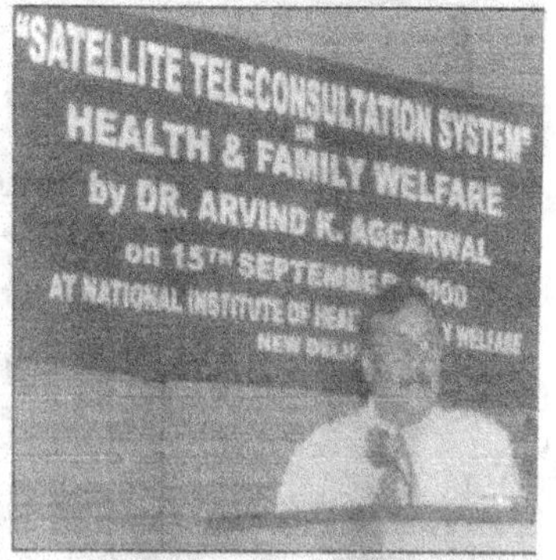

समय की बरबादी, आने जाने का खर्च और परेशानी अलग। टेलीमेडीसिन इसलिए आई.टी. का एक जादू है। इससे भारत जैसे देश को फायदा उठाना चाहिए।

प्रश्न : सूचना प्रौद्योगिकी इतनी महंगी चीज है। इसमें संचार की लागत भी आएगी। टेलीमेडीसिन सेंटर बनाने में पूंजी लागत भी होगी। पूंजी की अपनी कीमत होती है। इस सबको देखते हुए यह इतनी सस्ती कैसे हो सकती है?

उत्तर : हमारी जांचें सब डिजिटल मशीनें से होती हैं। इनमें न फिल्म खर्च होती है, न केमीकल। ई.सी.जी. भी पेपरलैस। हमें जांच के लिए बड़े स्टाफ और प्रयोगशाला की जरूरत नहीं। असल में यह सब टेक्नोलॉजी का कमाल है। आप जानते हैं कि पहले ए-4 साइज के एक कागज की विदेश फैक्स करने में 50 रुपये खर्च हो जाते थे और आज ई-मेल से उसे भेजने में न के बराबर खर्च आता है। टेलीमेडीसिन की प्रणाली चूंकि संचार इमेजिंग तथा डाटा स्टोरिंग आदि चीजों में किफायती प्रदान करती है तथा डाक्टरों के समय की भी बचत करती है, इसलिए यह इतनी सस्ती संभव है। इसमें सीधा-सादा गणित और अर्थशास्त्र है।

प्रश्न : लोग आम तौर पर अपने फैमिली डाक्टर को पसंद करते हैं। टेलीमेडीसिन के मामले में न जाने किस डाक्टर के पल्ले पड़ जाएं? परिचित चेहरा विहीन प्रणाली में कौन भरोसा जताएगा?

उत्तर : यह सब आदत की बात है। मुझे याद है, बचपन में हमारे यहां ग्वाला दूध लेकर आता था। मां कभी-कभी उससे शिकायत करती

VXL Instruments ties up with foreign firm

VXL Instruments Limited, a leading manufacturer of computer terminals and monitors with manufacturing facilities at Bangalore has tied up with Esprit Systems, Inc., San Jose, USA. Esprit Systems, Inc. is part of the ADI Group of Taiwan.

ADI is known worldwide as a major player in the IT industry, specializing in design, manufacture and sales of computer products and peripherals on a worldwide basis.

IT companies of ADI Group have manufacturing plants in Taiwan, Thailand and US, employing over 1200 employees, assets over US $ 103 million and sales of US $ 500 million. The IT products include colour monitors of various sizes. The company also offers various types of monochrome and colour terminals. ADI plants produce and sell over 2 million colour monitors every year. Among the IT companies in the ADI group is Esprit Systems Inc., USA, pioneers in computer terminal industry.

ADI products are sold and serviced globally through their offices in the USA, Taiwan and Thailand. Esprit Systems Inc., San Jose, USA, pioneers in computer terminal industry belong to the ADI group. Esprit range includes ASCII/ ANSI and special purpose terminals. Esprit have tied up with VXL Instruments Limited, Bangalore, for supply of 14" monochrome terminals. Under this arrangement VXL is to supply 50,000 terminals to Esprit. The terminals designed by VXL instruments, to be sup-

Health care round the clock

Sevati Devi Memorial Hospital & Advanced Institute of Medical Sciences & Research, New Delhi, plans to provide global health expertise for the global health care round the clock besides providing world standard emergency treatment at the door steps of the patients within a few minutes. Instead of patients going to the hospital, the hospital will go to the patient.

The project envisages to create a chain of 20,000 medical kiosks in the first phase all over India.

With the help of the video conference a patient in its hospital can get advice from the best doctors in their respective facilities in India and abroad, through the satellite channels.

Supposing the opinion of one specialist is not enough and a second opinion is required, without going abroad immediately by just turning the knobs, a second opinion from another world renowned specialist, from another corner of the world can be sought.

In case the opinions are conflicting, then simultaneous conference of all the specialists can be arranged, who will have the complete physical and bio-medical data of the patient before them and will be seeing the patient and discussing with each other, to reach the final conclusion. Hence, the patient without wasting time, money and without having to travel abroad will get the world's latest and best treatment at heavily reduced cost.

Just like 'Mother Dairy Booths' in Delhi the aid will be available to the patient within easy reach. These kiosks will work around the clock and will be equipped with emergency treatment facilities. Just by using an insurance card or a credit card or another similar instrument, a patient will have access to the hospital's central computerised OPD and can consult doctors in the language of his choice. Professionally qualified staff will always be available kiosks to provide emergency treatment and to do physical examination of the patient.

Medical kiosks can be built in every locality and will be easily approachable to the patients. The charges will be standardised. These could be paid through insurance card, credit cards and instruments like telephones cards issued in foreign countries. A general practitioner will have access to specialist/super specialists and will be able to offer better standard of treatment.

Once a person has franchise for a 'kiosk' at one place, he can use this franchise, to shift to the kiosk at any other place in case he changes his place of work or his family shifts. So it will suit the floating population of professionals.

The remotest parts of our country will be connected through the satellite channel. Since every kiosk will be watched on video continuously, the services rendered will be continuously under supervision and strictly controlled for quality to be provided as per present standards.

Since there are no cash transactions taking place, the question of fleecing the patient and over charging will be over.

Ambulances equipped with video conference facilities, including qualified medical staff and facilities for emergency treatment, will be placed at strategic points in Greater Noida and Delhi, from where they can reach the patient immediately within five to ten minutes. For the above project technical know how has been proposed by World Health Organisation (Through ECRI) on non-profit sharing basis.

Self-employment job vistas open to over 1,50,000 medical para-medical professionals. A state-of-the-art Rs. 300 crore hospital at Greater Noida will bring world-class heath care right to your doorstep.

CRB Caps posts excellent results

CRB Capital Markets Limited, the leading financial services power house has posted excellent results for the year ended March 31, 1995. According to 407 crore which makes it the second largest private sector finance company. Income from operations has gone up by 252.93 per cent, profit before depreciation and services industry.

The company has operations in bill discounting and corporate funds management, merchant

Technotelemedicine invited to join UNESCO in its Gujrat project

In a recent development, UNESCO has invited Techno Telemedicine and Telehealth Care Ltd., to join them in their Gujrat project. Techno Telemedicine and Telehealth Care Ltd., intends to provide world class healthcare to common man at low cost, home monitoring ser-

vices to cardiac, asthamtic, diabetic, hypertension patients, global consultation at patients' bed side without patient having to travel abroad, guidance to surgeons in remote areas. The whole system is an attempt to make healthcare industry as a organised sector.

Director General Health Services, Haryana, Dr P L Jindal who came to see the telemedicine technology show at Bristol Hotel Gurgaon said, "This will bring a revolution in the Healthcare Industry." These remarks are

Hanumanthappa, superintendant, General Hospital, Jaya Nagar Bangalore wrote in his report submitted to the health minister Dr A B Malakka Reddy said "this programme will change the face of healthcare Karnataka if implemented."

Dr A B Malakka Reddy (health

minister of Karnataka) who visited the office of Technotelemedicine in Gurgaon wanted to know everything in detail and asked Dr Aggarwal to demonstrate the technology in detail and spent almost three and a half hours. He tried all digital equipment on himself and learnt their use.

At the technology show organised by Technotelemedicine last month, eminent guests from health industry were Shri G Madhavan principal secretary health, Haryana, Dr P L Jindal Director

Dr K C Jain Civil Surgeon Haryana, Dr Abeykoon and Ms Iyotsna Chikersal from World Health Organisation, Shri Ashok sharma from UNESCO, Director Health Services and his team from Pondicherry, Director General Health Services Goa, Dr Meera Singh and Dr Bishwas from Indian Council of Medical Research just to name a few.

Technotelemedicine showed a live open heart operation from National Hospital Norway and Robotic surgery. SINTEF telecom and Informatics CEO, addressed the audience through video conference. Larsen and Toubro representative said they are supporting the project.

On 18th July, Shri Surjeet Banerjee, Principal Secretary Health UP Government had invited

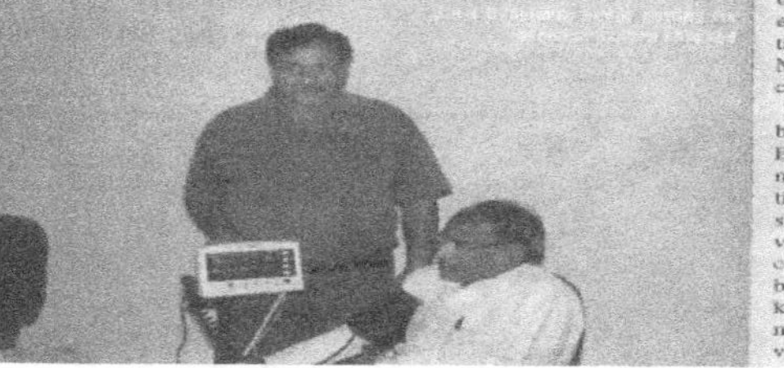

Dr Arvind Aggarwal for presentation at the secretariat Lucknow. The meeting was attended by Shri D P Misra, Secretary Health, Shri Yogesh Kumar, Secretary Medical Education and other special secretaries, joint secretaries. Dr Arvind Aggarwal was also scheduled to give a presentation at Bhubneshwar (Orissa) on the invitation of the Principal Secretary Health Meena Gupta, but the same got cancelled due to floods in the

State.

The project shall change the face of healthcare in the nation by setting up National network of Satellite Medical Centres to provide world class healthcare at low affordable cost. A patient shall be able to get entire examination, basic standard investigations of blood, urine, stool and ECG and specialised consultation for a flat fees of Rs 50. It offers better paid employment to doctors as franchisees with continued medical education, secured business opportunity with high returns to Satellite Medical Centers franchisees and channel partners.

Pharmaceutical companies shall be benefited heavily. Alpharma, a European pharmaceutical company has shown interest in participation. Each Satellite Medical Center shall have a chemist shop to provide standardised medicines at low cost the patients as bulk buying, bulk packing, elimination of marketing cost shall reduce cost of medicines for patients while providing bulk business to pharma-

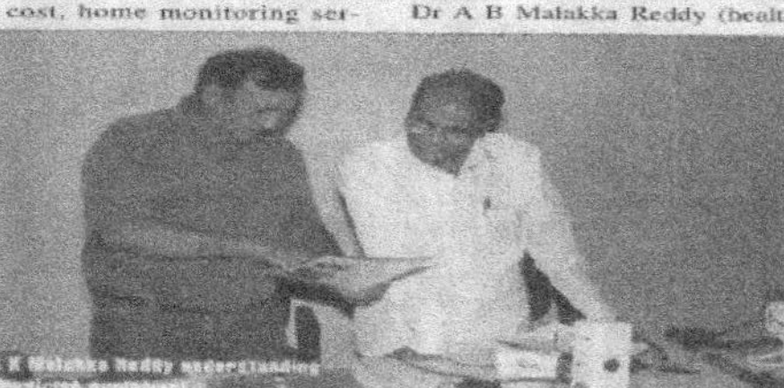

EXPRESS Healthcare Management

India's First Newspaper For The Healthcare Business

Vol. 2 No.10   1-15 June 2001   20 + 8 pages   Rs. 25.00

Mega telemedicine project to offer nationwide healthcare

GIREESH CHANDRA PRASAD G I
New Delhi

TECHNO Telemedicine and Telehealthcare, a Delhi-based company, is floating an ambitious telemedicine project linking 15,000 medical centers across more than ten states. The project aims at providing telemedicine services to patients at a payment of just Rs 50.

The Rs 9,000-crore mega project entails participation (in terms of equity and expertise) from internationally renowned institutions such as Sintef University, Riks Hospital, and Norway and Telenor - a reputed telecom company.

The project, conceptualised on the hub and spokes model, will have an Internet hub centre at Gurgaon, Haryana duly linked to Satellite Medical Centres (SMCs) spread across the country. The Government of Haryana has already granted 20 acres of land to set up the central hub.

More than ten state governments including Assam, Manipur, Meghalaya, Goa, Karnataka, Andhra Pradesh, Madhya Pradesh, Jammu & Kashmir as well as Haryana have already agreed to take part in the project and provide necessary support. States like Punjab, Himachal Pradesh and Rajasthan are expected to join the project soon. Techno Telemedicine is soon to hold presentations before the state authorities of Orissa, West Bengal, Kerala and Rajasthan.

Impressed by the project, the Indian Council of Medical Research (ICMR) has already recommended the Union Ministry of Health and Family Welfare to support the pilot project in Gurgaon. Dr Arvind Aggarwal, CMD, Techno Telemedicine & Telehealthcare told EHM in an interview. Among the states, the Government of Goa has already made a budget allocation to implement the project in the state. Dr Aggarwal expects WHO participation in the project soon.

Once the planned 15,000 Satellite Medical Centres, spread across 600 districts, are linked to the hub, patients can just walk in any of these SMC and avail all basic investigations, including blood, urine, ECG and X-Ray. The SMC will record the details about the patient in the form of an audio-visual text file and will be sent to the consultants at the hub. The patients can thus avail treatment as per the advice of the consultants at the central hub through the doctors at the SMC. The history of the patient will be kept at the hub and can be retrieved from any of the SMC. The project will highly reduce the cost of treatment, reduce unnecessary reference to various hospitals and standardise treatment.

The project also aims to provide home monitoring system employing specialised gadgets connected to the Net, global consultancy facility and expert guidance to doctors at rural areas for performing surgery. The technical support and network management will be provided by Telenor.

The Asia Pacific Centre for Transfer of Technology (APCTT) has already signed an agreement with us to commercialise this technology to neighbouring countries, Dr Aggarwal informed.

Hinduja Hospital to offer home-based chemotherapy

SOUMYA V
Mumbai

IN a month or two Hinduja Hospital will trail blaze the concept of giving chemotherapy to patients at home. The Hospital will send its trained team of professionals to offer services at the patients' doorsteps.

Speaking to EHM, Dr Asha Kapadia, medical oncologist, informed, "It is too premature to give details. It is not structured as yet." She added that though there are consultants giving chemotherapy at home and she has herself done it before, delivering it as a team is a different ball game altogether. "A different method of operation has to be followed. We have lots of home work to do," Dr Kapadia says. A lot of aspects like insurance and medico-legal need to be considered, she added.

Home care in US includes nursing, physiotherapy, chemotherapy, parenteral, nursing, rehabilitation and more. "In fact, in US, the home care personnel are on beepers so that they are available all the time," says Dr Kapadia. Though we have a long way to go before this is home care institutions are set up and this is achieved, Hinduja's step is certainly in the right direction.

Chapter 12

THE MECHANISM

Every Digital Medical Centre (DMC) is powered by a digital infrastructure. It is a profit-making unit - a business where any person or entity can invest for returns on the investment, just like individuals invest in bank fixed deposits.

Working on the sa me principle, a resident welfare association or a builder or a corporate entity such as a bank or business venture can invest in Digital Medical Centre(s). The DMCs are operated by different service providers with Doctor(s) as franchisee partner .

Now, besides the obvious democratic nature of such a set-up, what makes this healthcare delivery mode especially attractive is that the franchisee partners (physicians/doctors) can *work from anywhere* (at any DMC) and earn much beyond what their present terms of service (whether public or private) will allow. In addition, the franchisee partner experiences *a greater volume of available time at his/her disposal.* Especially in times of a sudden family engagement or an impromptu vacation, the franchisee partner will experience the real benefits of such a system.

For instance, say, I am a franchisee partner (Doctor). My wife who is a Doctor in a government hospital, has just been transferred to a different city. Instead of trying to get her transfer cancelled, I can now join her wherever she is posted, and work at any nearby DMC where there is a vacancy (the internet-based App auto-updates the vacancy slots so the franchisee partner may book a slot).

To commence treatment, the franchisee partner (Doctor) can avail either options - *DMC Clinic* (Out Patient Department/OPD) or *Doctor-at-Home* (Home Visit). The DMC Clinic functions like an Outdoor Patient Department (or OPD) where patients may either 'walk-in' or fix an appointment through the App or the helpline number.

Since both the DMC Clinic or 'Doctor at Home' performs the same functions with differences only in the matter of conduction of diagnostic tests for the 'Home Visit', one may understand the process through a close look into the ' *Doctor-at-Home*' option.

Doctor-at-Home (Home Visit)
On receiving a patient request for home visit (through routed call), the Doctor's digital account dashboard will automatically execute a booking request through a partner app-based cab platform (Ola/Uber/other). This helps the doctor reach the patient faster and hassle-free (the payment for the ride is borne by the digital platform).

At the *onsite* the Doctor shall examine the patient,

and may conduct regular blood investigations (including HB, TLC, DLC, Blood Sugar, Liver function tests, Kidney function tests, Lipid profile, etc.) and EchoCardiogram or ECG with instant results. Should the patient require specialised consultation, say with a Cardiologist or Neurologist, the Doctor-at-home arranges the same at the patient's bedside instantaneously.

Patient's audio-video-text EMR is shared with the Specialist and the latter's advice for further line of treatment is followed. The prescription is routed through the digital platform to the nearest pharmacy for doorstep delivery to the patient.

The Doctor-at-home (visiting doctor) is entitled to a fixed income per home visit inclusive of investigations. Besides, such a Doctor also accrues a 33 % share of the Specialist-Consultant's fees.

With regard to Consultant fees - every Consultant, exercising due discretion, 'sets' his/her fees. This is for two reasons. Fees for specialised consultation(s) cannot be pre-determined or 'imposed'. Second, this system allows the market forces to act freely, ensuring every Consultant is enthused to provide the best service so s/he may emerge as the preferred Consultant.

The patients realise the direct benefit of zero waiting-time through consultations at home or at the DMC. In cases where X-ray, MRI or Ultrasound or CT scan is advised, the patient shall be required to visit the DMC for imaging or diagnostic services. This is because most X-ray or MRI machines are bulky and require a controlled environment.

The X-ray or MRI so obtained is attached to the EMR in the patient file and can be retrieved for review and reference by the clinical expert as and when required. Similarly, specialised investigations may also be ordered or outsourced from a laboratory operating outside the DMC and such laboratory shall upload the reports or slides etc. on the patient's dashboard towards the necessary assessment.

In the digital diagnostics system, results are available within a maximum time duration of 2 to 3 minutes. This results in instant diagnosis and prescription by the physician, effectively eliminating the 2-visit system and waiting-time, expediting the commencement of treatment and putting the patient on the 'fast(est) track' to healthcare and recovery.

THIS IS THE MOST **COMPREHENSIVE , SELF SUSTAINING & REVOLUTIONARY HEALTHCARE DELIVERY MODEL** ANYWHERE IN THE WORLD.

With **FAR - REACHING EFFECTS.**

* * *

BIDDING ADIEU to the "2-VISITS" SYSTEM

In the conventional healthcare delivery system, the patient's first visit will usually proceed as follows. The Doctor hears and records the 'Patient History', then examines the patient and thereafter, prescribes treatment based on the symptoms or prescribes investigations. After a few days, say a week later, the patient comes back with the reports. The Doctor will now check the reports and adjust or start the treatment, as the case may be. This, at the minimum, is a "2-visits" treatment process.

This results in a time lapse before treatment can be commenced. And the element of *time* may be especially critical in the case of serious maladies requiring instant medical intervention. Besides, the patient must do 'rounds' of diagnostic centres or laboratories for the conduction of the tests, collection of reports etc. In the process, the patient undergoes unplanned expenditures for tests and transportation and finding a helper (adding up to a several thousands), besides the psychological costs of going through hitherto unknown diagnostic processes. And the added cost of waiting period and a further deterioration of the patient's physical and mental state.

* * *

MINIMAL COST HEALTHCARE

In the proposed system, all routine and specialised investigations can be done through the DMC. This helps in strict quality control with respect to diagnostic services, ensuring all quality parameters are met universally across the country/world, as the case may be. Furthermore, the use of uniform digital devices helps in trimming down the costs. Add to it, the effective elimination of wasteful use of valuable resources such as paper, films and chemicals through the use of digital diagnostic records - and costs are brought down further.

This reduction in costs translates into direct benefits to the patient, who needs to pay a flat sum of, say . Rs 200, as total cost of the investigations, including most of the special investigations of blood and urine that may be prescribed. (Note: In case of special investigations beyond those that are covered by the system, the same will incur additional direct payment by the patient).

Thus, the actual diagnostic cost beyond the per patient stipulation of Rs 200 is absorbed by the system, effectively rendering healthcare services free for most patients. This is made possible through the vast number of beneficiaries who are using the system at any given point in time, where the individual patient stands to gain. This innovation of a standard cost/patient shall ensure medical attention to patients who might otherwise find it unaffordable to benefit from quality healthcare and hence fall outside the healthcare network of the state. This also renders healthcare services more popular and helps *bring every person under the umbrella of a robust 24/7 Universal Healthcare system*

With regard to the medical team, the revenue generated through the franchisee partner (Doctor) fees plus commission (at 33%) from the Consultant-Specialist comprises a very competitive remuneration for the Doctor.

With regard to the DMC, every DMC will charge token commissions from the doctors and the consultants. Add to it, the revenue from all the diagnostic services, and the digital healthcare delivery system is self-equipped to absorb transportation charges and investigations' charges, thereby rendering healthcare services unprecedentedly inexpensive and unhinderingly accessible to all patients irrespective of their geographies or socio-economic conditions through advanced digital technology.

* * *

GET WELL *SOONEST*

This automated system of healthcare delivery rules out aggravation of the malady by effectively obliterating the time lapse between the physician's prescription for diagnostic tests and the actual tests and communication of their results. Here, the diagnosis and prescription is immediate, preventing the malady from lingering on while reports of the inve stigations are awaited.

This digital system cuts down the examination time per person, for all visits, especially those after the first visit. In the '2-visits' system , the first visit/consultation would normally be around 8 to 10 minutes while the second visit would last about 4 to 6 minutes; so, the total consultation time would be approximately 14 minutes.

In the new model, the total time for the actual consultation can be really short (close to 2 minutes) as the Physician/Consultant can *see* the complete patient information in a well-organised manner, in one go. Also, once the case history of the patient is recorded and the results of various diagnostic tests uploaded on the patient dashboard, all subsequent consultations can be conducted most effectively without wastage in terms of time. This eventually results in optimal efficiency (by upto 7 - 8 times) and the opportunity of reaching treatment to a greater number of patients in the same amount of time.

Optimising wellness treatment in the least amount of time, this model puts the patient back on his/her feet expeditiously, reducing both th e cost of treatment and the loss in work days due to illness.

* * *

***INNOVATIVE* SOLUTION TO TACKLE RESOURCE CRUNCH**

This model is India's answer to the paucity crisis of healthcare professionals, especially Specialists. Going by reports that estimate anywhere around 200000 active consultants in India today, the new healthcare model powered through a digital infrastructure will result in improving their productivity by 7 -8 times, at the least. While this helps cut the cost-per-consultation by 1/7th - 1/8th for every patient; it goes a long way in building accessibility to the best and most affordable healthcare service for the common man.

The 'production' period for new physicians and specialists roughly comprises 12 years, from start to finish. So, by the time a new specialist-consultant completes education and training to start 'practice'; roughly the same size of professionals is on the verge of retirement. This is revealed most tellingly through the statistics of the recent years which demonstrate that the 'net production' of healthcare professionals has remained, more or less, the same with only marginal growth in a few sectors.

Through the present innovation, however, our country shall not only resolve the dearth of trained professionals, but will be adequately well-equipped to export the healthcare services that are available in surplus to other nations. Also, in a trickle-down effect, availability of Specialists will effect a greater upgradation of healthcare services while reducing cost.

Add to this, India's emergence as a major exporter of healthcare services to the world, and we will not only help eliminate the global paucity of Specialists but also herald India's emergence as a leader in the healthcare sector (on the same lines as its emergence in the IT sector). Most importantly, even the last human being in the remotest village shall be able to access specialised and affordable healthcare. Instantly. 24 x 7.

***

TRANS-NATIONAL CONSULTATION

Assuming, a critical patient needs simultaneous consultation with five Specialist-Consultants:
One from Tata Cancer Hospital, Mumbai (India)
One from Medanta Hospital, Delhi (India)
One from National University Hospital, Singapore
One from King's College Hospital, London (UK) and
One from University of Tokyo Hospital, Tokyo (Japan) (where the incorporated auto-translation tool - a technological aid devised on the lines of the Japanese *Illi*, auto-starts to aid real-time speech communication during consultation) . The sophisticated in-built video/audio conferencing software will facilitate seamless global communication between the Doctor (at the DMC or visiting-at-home) and the Consultant(s) - Specialist(s).

Irrespective of the geographical location (across the world), the Consultant can speak with the patient in any intelligible language, even speak to the physician by the patient's side and/or conduct the examination through the aid of remote devices. This sophistication of customised care is unprecedented in the medical history of the world.

Patients can avail the best quality healthcare in an ethos of 'no travel costs, no visa and no repetitive cycles of physical visits to doctors. This implies that besides the zero waiting-time, patients are now able to access global healthcare without the worries of arranging for travelling, advance bookings an d other costly overheads. Thus, the patient can now actually and truly access global medical expertise from anywhere at any time.

So, while we cannot physically send the patient to five places in five different countries at the same time; the way I see it, we have devised a system that brings those five physicians from the different parts of the world together to the patient's bedside. It is like making available a global healthcare infrastructure to the patient's bedside in a complete paradigm shift from the erstwhile practice of queuing up for the physician's attention for hours on end.

* * *

*INSTANT AND ACCURATE*DIAGNOSIS

Chances of both misdiagnos is or missed diagnosis shall reduce by far through the latest digital devices used for investigations ofHb, blood sugar, ureaTLC that not only give accurate but also i nstant results. Similarly, results from digital devices t hat can do specialised tests instantly to gauge kidney function, liver function and lipid profile, are integrated into the patient's 'Health Records' dashboard. In addition, image-capturing devicesused in healthcare such as X-ray, MRI, CT scan, CT Angioplasty and Ultrasound, work compatibly with the PACS and Dicom plat form in the web-based environment.

All image reports achieved digitally as also the pictures from other investigations such as Pathology slides are directly uploaded in the patient EMR.

Whenever new information is added, it shall be tagged by the doctor ID and DMC code. In strict adherence to norms relating to non - tampering of medical data, the system is de vised such that information can be added but cannot be altered or deleted. Any subsequent alteration in the information may be recorded through the same process as the adding of new information.

All data shall exist on cloud in encrypted format to maintain confidentiality. In a strategic innovation to ensure privacy and security of data, the medical records in audio-visual and text and video files (EMR) cannot be accessed without due authorisation.

This will have a phenomenal impact on the quality of diagnosis and by extension, the line of treatment. In turn, this will effect a true globalisation of healthcare where all the stakeholders benefit through the improvement in the delivery and quality of healthcare.

* * *

IMPARTIAL AND EFFECTIVE TREATMENT

The 'smart system' creates a model for objective assessment of the patient's progress. Several images of eye(s), ear or throat or the findings of the ECG, X-ray or other investigations can be instantly viewed side-by-side and compared in the minutest details and most accurate shades of colour.

This feature is especially useful as currently we largely rely on the subjective method for assessing improvements or deterioration in the patient's health condition. For instance, in response to a physician's query of *How are you now?* the patient may, at times, give incorrect information deliberately, under the compulsion to prolong the hospital stay or for other reasons of concern, say, the issue of post-discharge care.

The single most important advantage of this system is that the Consultant has, at her/his disposal, a system that enables her/him to examine the patient directly or indirectly and/or view the diagnostic test reports himself/herself, thereby not depending upon the inference made by the primary physician. The objective nature of such clinical practice helps in generating a high degree of medical rigour at all levels.

For instance, turning back to the example mentioned earlier - the five different Specialist-Consultants from five different institutions (often spread across the globe) from the same or allied specialties examining this patient, need not depend upon half-baked, incomplete or incorrect inferences passed on by juniors or others. So, each one of them 'sees' different things and draws independent autonomous conclusions. The objectivity built into the system, helps the Specialist(s), at all times, to directly see, hear and analyse the information on the basis of their knowledge and experience and such independent, in-depth and impartial analysis directly benefits the patient.

GLOBAL HEALTHCARE DELIVERY SYSTEM

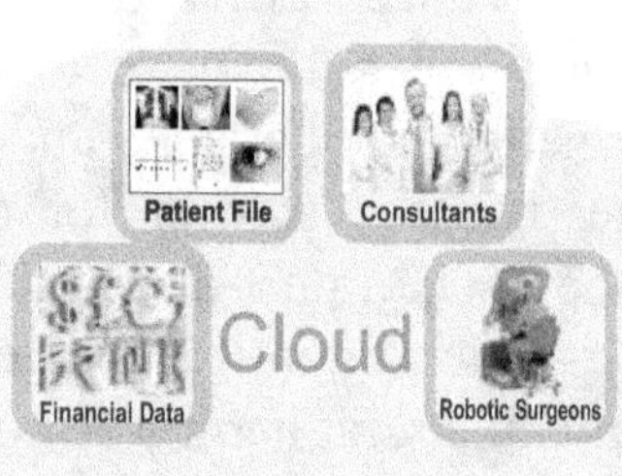

ONLINE SPEECH & TEXT TRANSLATION SYSTEM

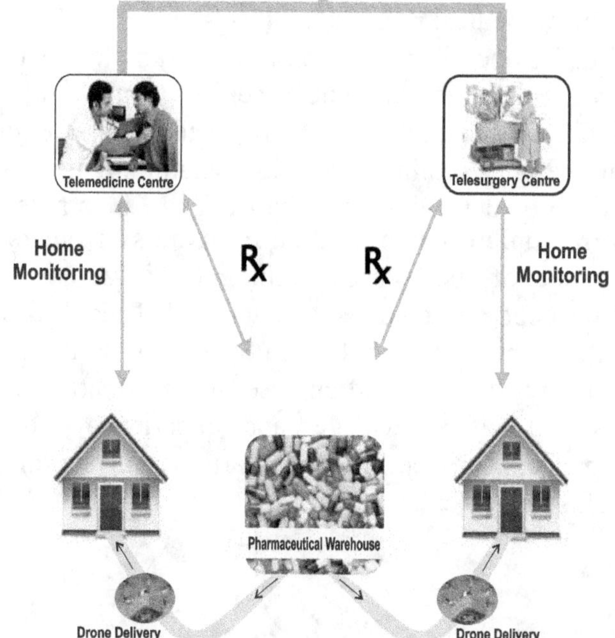

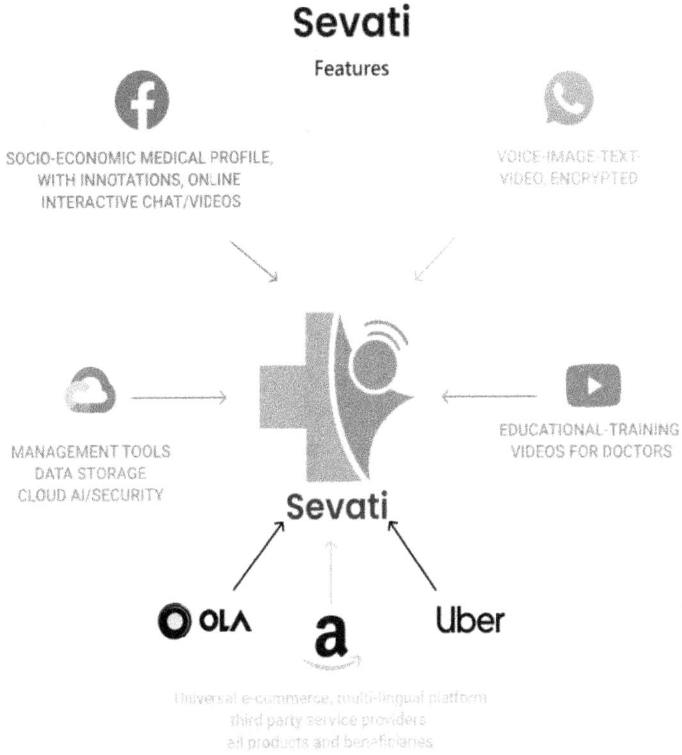

Sevati

Features

An IT based Global Healthcare Delivery System

A
One-of-its-kind
One-Stop Solution
ensuring
Universal Healthcare

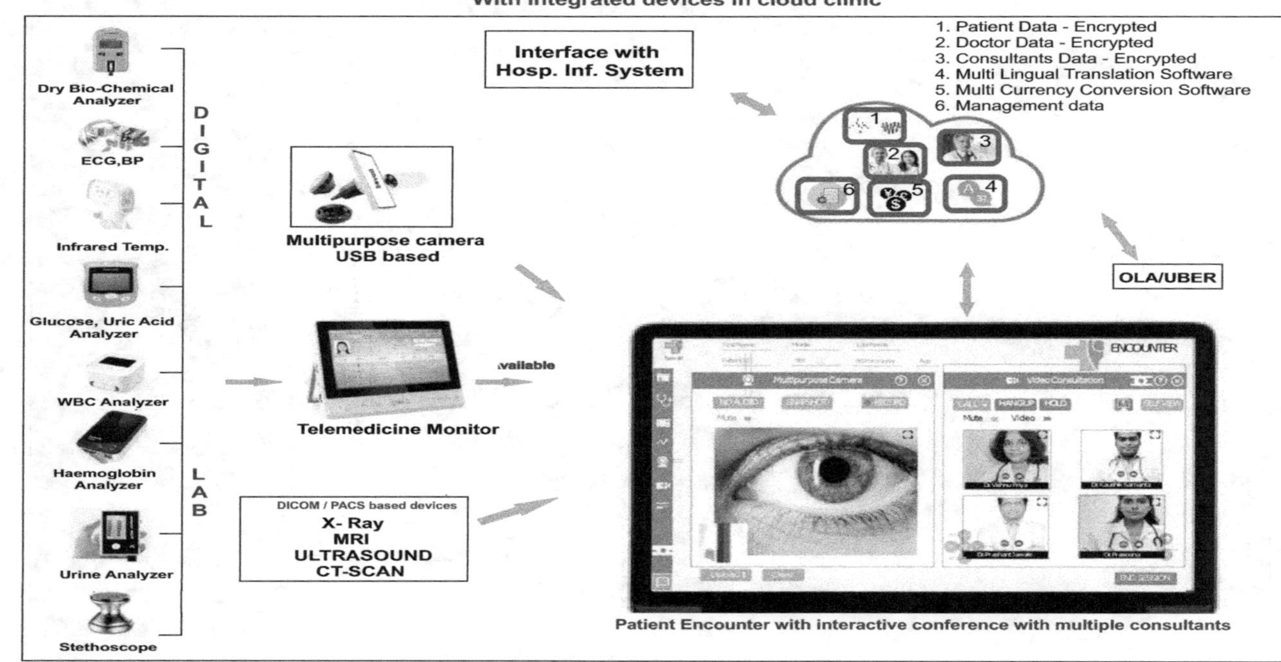

IT (CLOUD) BASED GLOBAL HEALTHCARE DELIVERY SYSTEM ©
With integrated devices in cloud clinic
Interface with Hosp. Inf. System
1. Patient Data - Encrypted
2. Doctor Data - Encrypted
3. Consultants Data - Encrypted
4. Multi Lingual Translation Software
5. Multi Currency Conversion Software
6. Management data
OLA/UBER
ENCOUNTER
Dry Bio-Chemical Analyzer
ECG,BP
Infrared Temp.
Glucose, Uric Acid Analyzer
WBC Analyzer
Haemoglobin Analyzer
Urine Analyzer
Stethoscope
DIGITAL
LAB
Multipurpose camera USB based
Telemedicine Monitor
Available
DICOM / PACS based devices
X- Ray
MRI
ULTRASOUND
CT-SCAN
Patient Encounter with interactive conference with multiple consultants

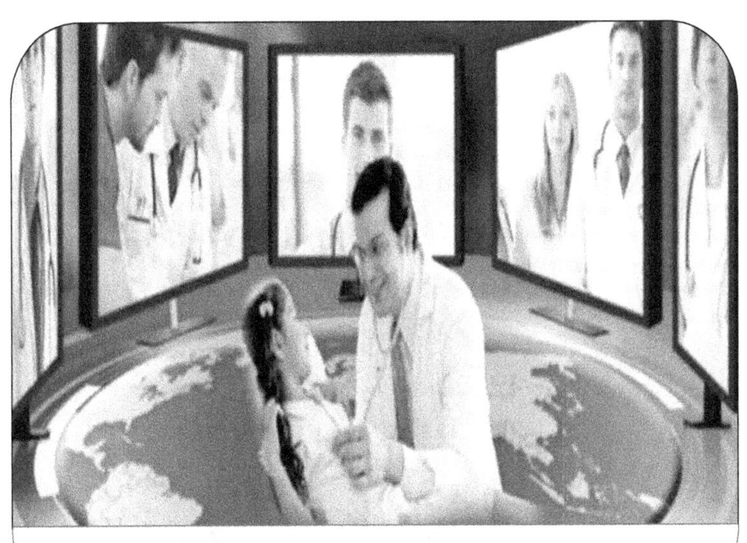

GLOBAL CONSULTATION SYSTEM

Chapter 13

THE TWO TRYSTS WITH TECHNOLOGY

The Elusive Telephone Line

The technological revolution today has made communication difficulties a thing of the past. For instance, when the mobile phone was first launched around 1994-95, it was a bulky set. I usually kept it in a special pouch that hung on the belt of my trousers to keep it in place without the distraction of dangling.

Today, an 'App' (think *WhatsApp*) that can be installed within a minute on our cellphones, has changed it all, drastically revolutionising the world of communication from the simple voice-based calls through a dial-up wired landline phone and receiver (this was much before the mobile phones pushed the landlines out of our drawing rooms). A time when it was difficult to get through a call from South Delhi to Chandni Chowk (famous market area in old Delhi) and a call outside the city (we called it a 'trunk-call' then!) needed to be routed through an "exchange" that would take anything upto a few days to connect one to friends or family staying outside the city.

Besides, the phone network hadn't been laid out in very many places in the first place, thereby making it difficult to acquire a phone connection on a landline device. I remember making an application for a landline phone connection which was expected to be installed in 6 months for Rs. 10000. Back in 1981. And this was typical of the rest of the world, too. I recall from my time in Hungary - when I first opened our Export office there, my landlady had been waiting for the landline for 7 years! They had planted the underground cable network line upto the door but now she was waiting for them to bring it inside the house!

First Brush with the FAX Machine!

While studying at the Medical College in Shimla, it would be extremely handy to have photocopies of important readings or reference material in preparation for writing research papers. However, there was not a single photocopy machine in all of Shimla. So, we'd normally travel to Chandigarh where there were a few photocopy shops, lugging about a dozen journals and books!

In Chandigarh, the photocopiers were very bulky and the process painfully slow. I remember dozing off at the photocopy shop to the mechanical sound of the xerox machine emitting copies of each page of the journal through half the evening.

During my maiden visit to Europe (1983), I travelled to Stockholm in Sweden. And while I was there, I went to a photocopier shop one evening. I wished to buy a Canon photocopier for my office as it was not yet available in India.

I walked into the Canon showroom, casting an appreciative glance around at the vast collections of cameras, lenses, sc anners and printers, neatly displayed row after row on the white marble surface. The owner of the shop - a kindly looking bespectacled man came out from behind the counter and smiled. When I told him why I was there, he asked me why I wanted to buy a Canon copier. I told him I was in the garment export business and the photocopier was needed for my office use.

The thick eyebrows just above his spectacles furrowed in thought as he put up a hand to slightly adjust the frame of his glasses.

"Let me show you one more device . . . which could be even more useful for your business," he said, walking me towards the counter where he had been seated earlier. And he showed me- theFAX MACHINE!

On the office desk, there were two fax machines installed one in fr ont of another.

For demo, he typed my name on a sheet of white paper and sent the paper through one of the machines and sure enough, a copy of it came out from the other!

I had neither seen, and truth be told, not even heard the word 'FAX' until this moment.

He explained the utility of such a device particularly for my office - how I could instantly transfer designs to my buyers and suppliers. Across towns, cities and even countries.

But I had never seen anything like this, leave alone the question of putting it to use. He was genuinely surprised that we didn't have it in India. But he totally persuaded me about the merits of buying the FAX machine. I was upbeat about the technology and very keen to buy one, too but did not know if our telephone network in India was compatible with FAX transmission.

So, I said, "I shall buy. . .*provided* it works in India." He agreed to give me a demo by sending a page to India and getting it back from there with something mentioned on it to show a response.

Unlike in India, post offices in Sweden are very resourceful. He spoke to the Post office in Stockholm to check if they could connect to a FAX number in India. May be in the Swedish embassy?

However, not a single fax number for India was found, and nobody had ever heard anything about any such communication. So, despite our best intent, I couldn't be sure whether the Fax machine would work back home.

As if reading my thoughts, he insisted, "If it does not work, you can bring it back and I will refund your money."If it did work, however, he proposed to partner with me in the business so we could jointly launch the Fax machine in India, promising me the Canon agency for the whole of India.

At about 12000 USD or Rs 1.25 lacs (1 USD was about 10 INR then), it was quite expensive at the time. I left it at that . . . I did not buy the Fax machine then.

* * *

Three months later, somebody told me that a business centre named Chawla Reprographics in Nehru Place (a commercial hub in South Delhi) has installed a FAX machine. My buyer representative Paola was due to come to India soon. I asked her to visit the Canon shop in Stockholm and bring a Fax machine for me. So, I had the second FAX machine in Delhi and amongst the first few in India.

Chapter 14

TAKE OFF!

First, there was the TELEX when I was growing up. It was a major means of sending text messages electronically. I remember when a Telex message would come, the whole building would reverberate. Nevertheless, it was the first instant transmission of word from one desk to another. Then came the FAX - it could transmit script and drawings. But it was gone too soon, almost as if pushed out the door by the Information Technology revolution. Soon enough, riding high on the IT wave, came the E-Mail. E-mail was instant digital transmissi on that spread digital communication wider and rendered it more versatile - an E-mail could transmit images, voices and videos besides text. However, we were still talking about heavy machines like TELEX, or a FAX machine or COMPUTERS.

Imagine the time when we used to pay Rs 100,000 rent/month for hiring 3 ISDN lines. The 2 Mbps mark was a dream. To be able to conduct real-time Video conferencing in the 2000s, we used to contemplate everything from ISDN lines, VSAT, transponders to satellites. Today, video conferencing is an app that comes incorporated in your e- mail! Bandwidth is free and wishfully used.

So, at the dawn of the new millennium, *the Idea to Universalise Healthcare* took its place on the policy tables and health consortiums of the world, but it could not take wings. Primarily because it was still too early and we had not woken up to the concept of affordable remote communication technology. All our efforts to translate *the Idea* into a solution and implement it on the ground came to a halting and heart-breaking standstill, for want of adequate broadband and storage technology. Time and again. We could not execute the Project because ofthe non-viability of the existing technology in relation to

- Broadbandand
- Data storage [14]

Very fortunately (I fully recognise that not all inventors will live to see their discoveries implemented on the ground), the technological limitations no longer remain, and today we can implement what we could not back in 2000. I find us in a space and a time where technology has matured enough to allow *this Idea* to germinate, this most loved brainchild to see the light of the day. And flourish.

28 years ago, the *Idea to Universalise Healthcare* across populations and geographies was a dream, often dismissed as a far-fetched vision. But not so today. In our 'trunk call' days, could we have anticipated reaching out instantly through *WhatsApp*? Even as I write, I know

that communications technology is advancing in leaps and bounds - becoming still faster, smoother and feature-rich. Besides, with 5G technology perched for a take-off, a new revolution in communication is in the offing, and almost as if signalling auspiciously, that now more than ever before the time is right to launch a more proficient model of how we communicate or deliver healthcare universally.

We're at the brink of a take-off . . .

* * *

And here we go . . . No! Stop!!

It was in the September of 1999, when I first realised the magnitude of the impact that *the Idea* could have on the world, primarily through the selection of my project ideation paper for presentation at the International Conference of G8 Countries in London. Much later, I realised that I was perhaps the only Indian representing my country at this consortium organised by the Royal Society of Medicine London and the American Telemedicine Service Providers Association or the ATSPA (I also received repeat invites in 2000 and 2001). Now, this made for a great space for sharing ideas and innovations amongst like-min ded collaborators. And it was here that I met Bob Phillips.

InBob,I have a friend and a brother - no less because he shares my obsession with **the Idea** and will be my partner-in-crime for the sake of the Project! It is indeed people like him who've helped sustain and strengthen my resolve to keep going, despite the many odds.

Bob was instrumental in bringing important

Norwegian companies as Consortium partners to the project. Amongst them were Telenor (we worked for two years together, holding several workshops in both India and Norway), who committed several hundred million dollars for the project, SINTEF (a large Norwegian IT Foundation) and Rikshospitalet (a part of Oslo University). Dag Christensen, working at the Telemedicine Department of Rikshospitalet, Oslo University Hospital, together with Prof. Eric Fosse, Head of the very advanced Department of Tele-Medicine and Robotic Surgery (working then to bring Robotics Surgery to the most far-flung geography through the 'single chip' technology) joined us with equal fervour. Back in the day, we were men on a united mission. To transform and universalise Healthcare Delivery system around the world.

What had held back Telemedicine in all our countries for the longest time was the traditional way of delivering healthcare. And it was this precise premise that united us despite our disparate geographies and varied socio-economic climes.

As Consortium partners, we worked hand-in-hand for almost 2 years, travelling together, making presentations to showcase the concept all over India. We received letters of interest from as many as 15 states of India. Particularly inspiring was our collaboration with the Konkan Railways. Our Memorandum of Understanding (MOU) with Konkan assigned us a plot at the Madgaon Rail Station towards developinga Digital Me dical Centre (DMC).

They even set up 3 rail wagons (2 with engines) for us, converting them into mobile DMCs to showcase the concept and its usefulness through live demo to the public,travelling from village to village.

Konkan Railways committed to setting up such

DMCs on all rail stations across India, should the proposed pilot project on the Konkan belt prove successful. Despite the great enthusiasm and Herculean efforts, the Project, heartbreakingly, could not be implemented as 'some bits of technology were still not invented'.

We stayed put. Several workshops were organised both in India and Norway where we discussed *the Idea* and its implementation challenges. Moving forward on those lines, we found ourselves tech partners in Tata Infotech and Larsen and Toubro!

Around the same time, I had the honour of discussing the Project at length with the very learnedDr. A P J Abdul Kalam (former President of India), who was at the time heading the Defence Research and Development Organisation (DRDO). Excited at the prospect of such a project being implemented in India, Dr. Kalam referred me to Dr . V S Ramamurthy (the then Secretary, Ministry of Science & Technology) with whom a series of brainstorming sessions ensued for a full week everyday from 10 am to 5 pm! We discussed, debated, reasoned and resolved that the Project would have a very real and revolutionary impact on the economy of India. Those were intense days with the best of intentions, but the technology - early in the dawn of the new millennium, was not mature enough yet to support its implementation.

"This project is futuristic. And we have to wait, some 20 years, till the technology matures and we implement it" ,Dr. V S Ramamurthy told me.

Little did I know then that his words would come true. And so precisely, too!

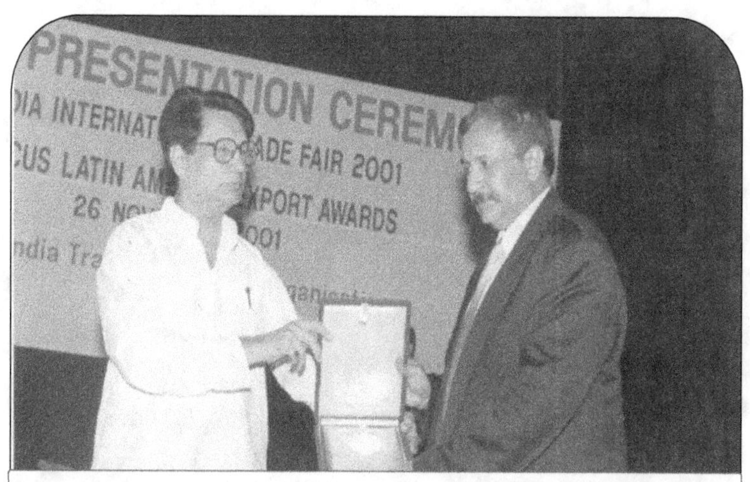

DR AGGARWAL BEING PRESENTED THE GOLD MEDAL BY THE UNION MINISTER SHRI.AJIT SINGH,FOR "BEST TECHNOLOGY INNOVATION" ON 26th NOVEMBER,2001

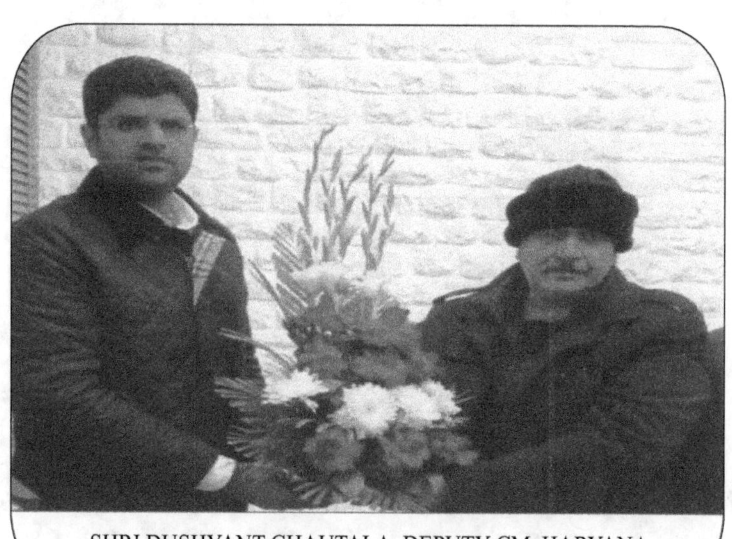

SHRI DUSHYANT CHAUTALA, DEPUTY CM, HARYANA
& DR. ARVIND AGGARWAL

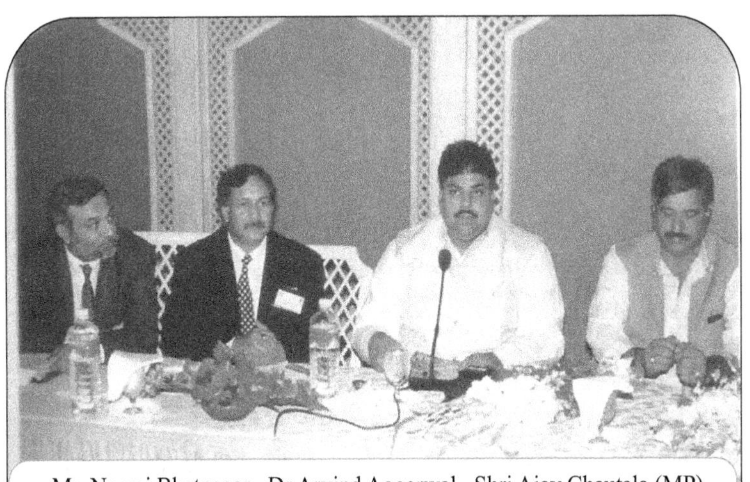

Mr. Neeraj Bhatnagar , Dr Arvind Aggarwal , Shri Ajay Chautala (MP)
& Shri S S Barwala (MP) on Our Function on 21 Dec 2000

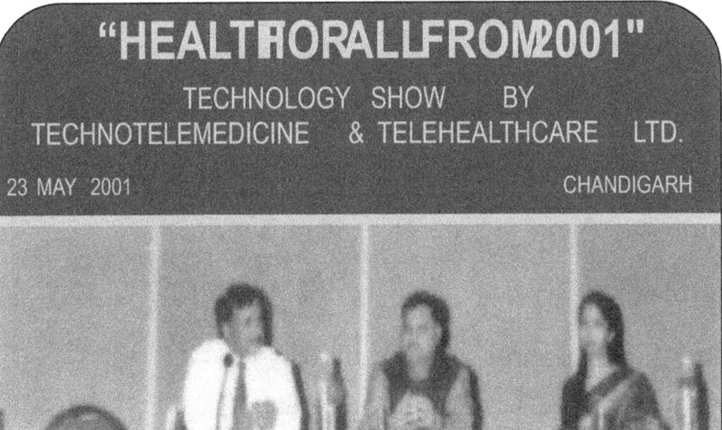

Dr Arvind Aggarwal , Shri J P Nadda(Health Minister- HP)
& Dr Meena Aggarwal at a conference in Chandigarh

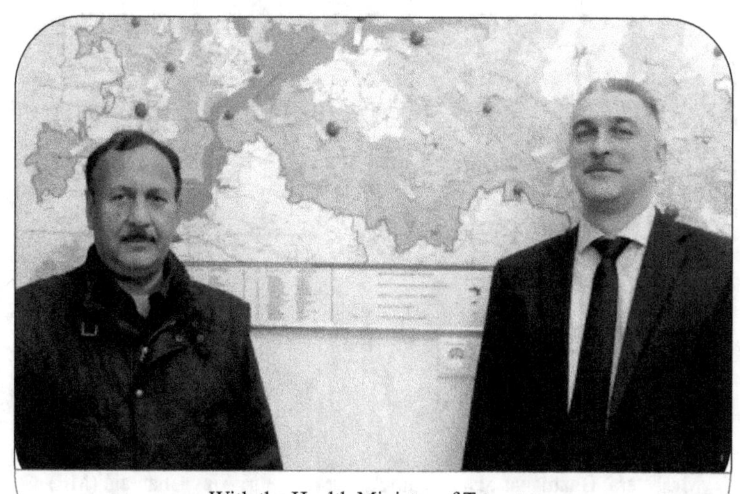

With the Health Minister of Tatarstan.
December 2018

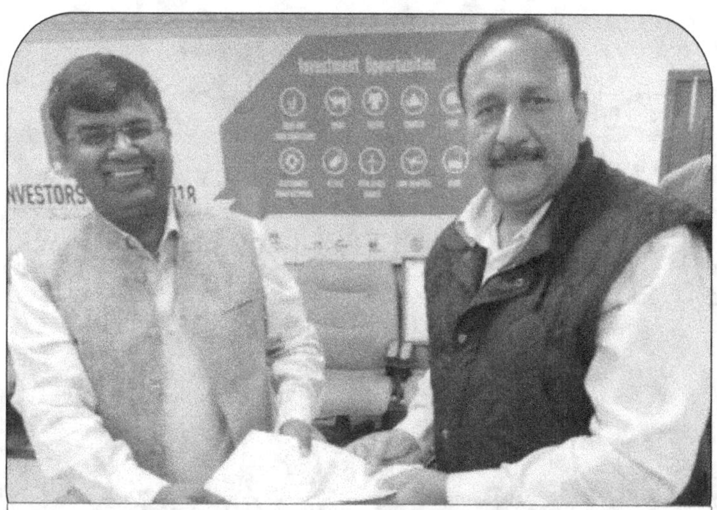

Signing the MOU to set up 300 DMCs!
With Shri Santosh Yadav (IAS), Secretary for Industry and
Development, Uttar Pradesh

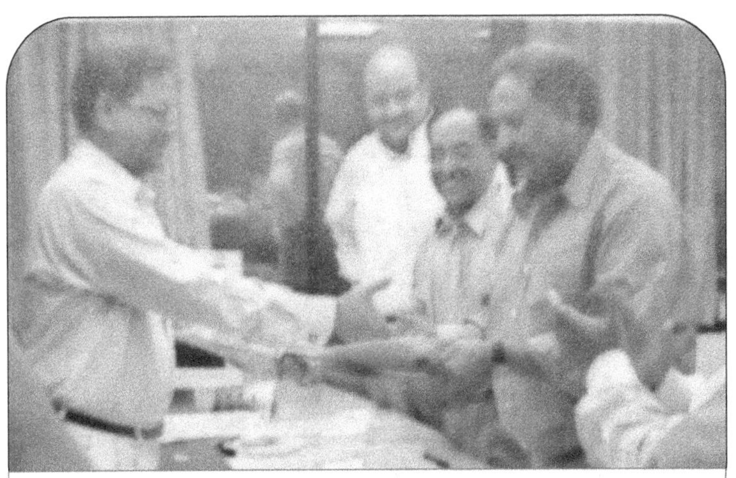

Signing Mou with MD,KRCL

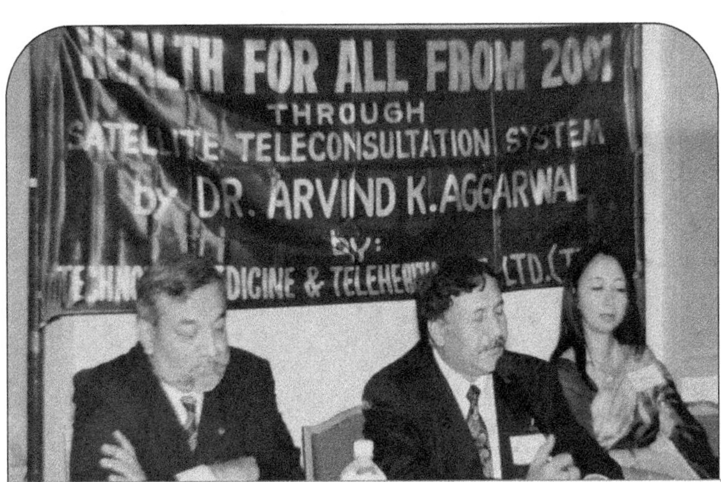

The Idea
Universal Healthcare: Instant, Remote, Affordable!

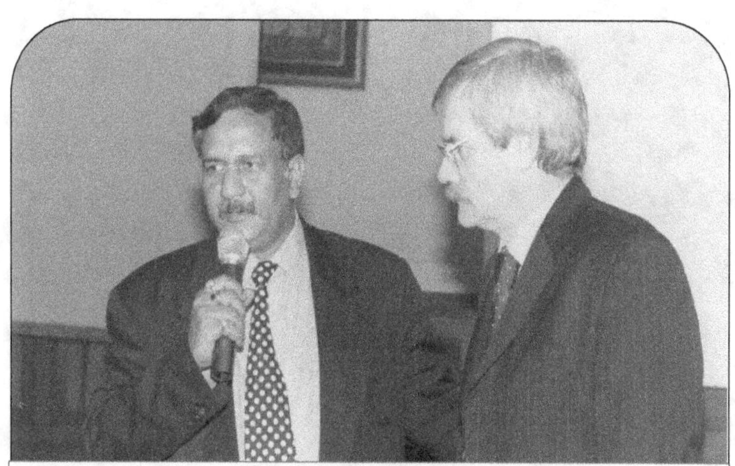

Men on the Mission!
Explaining the Viability of Remote Healthcare. In 2000.
Seen here with my friend Bob Phillips

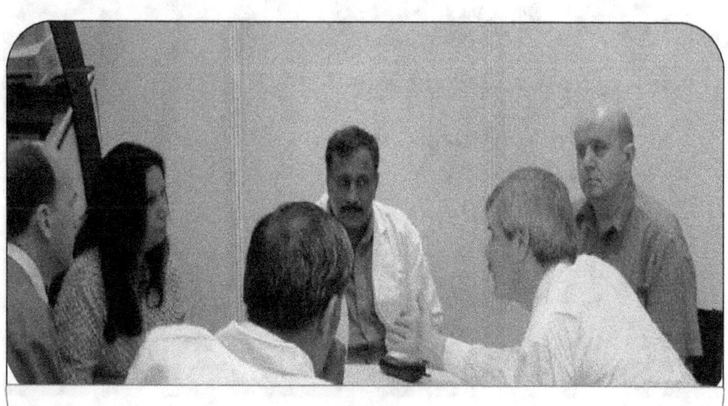

The Team at Work!
Left to Right: Bjorn, Pramila, Me, Dag and Robert

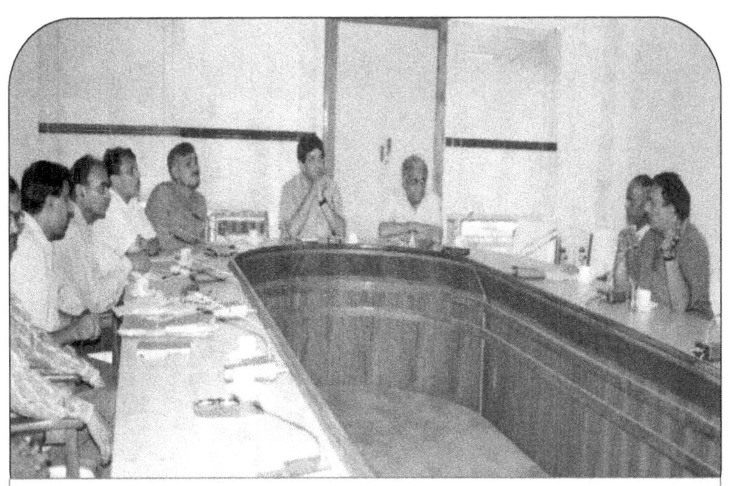

Explaining the Vision
At the Secretariat, UP Government (Lucknow) 2017

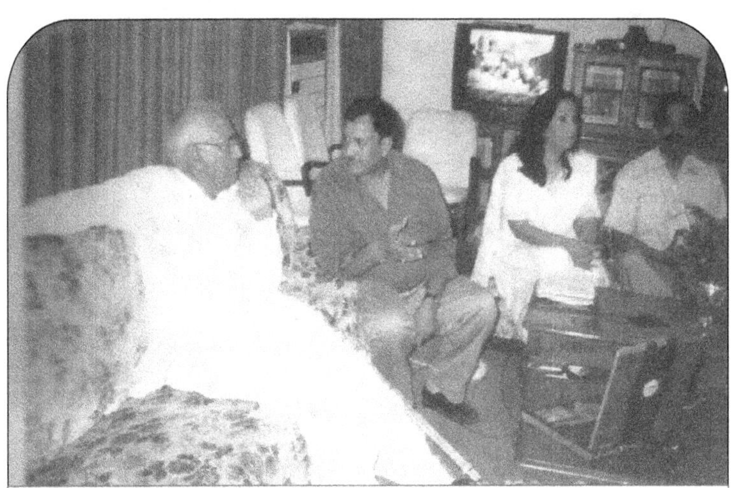

Dr. Arvind Aggarwal explaining the project to
Chief Minister Shri Om Prakash Chautala Chef Minister of Haryana
at his residence in Chandigarh

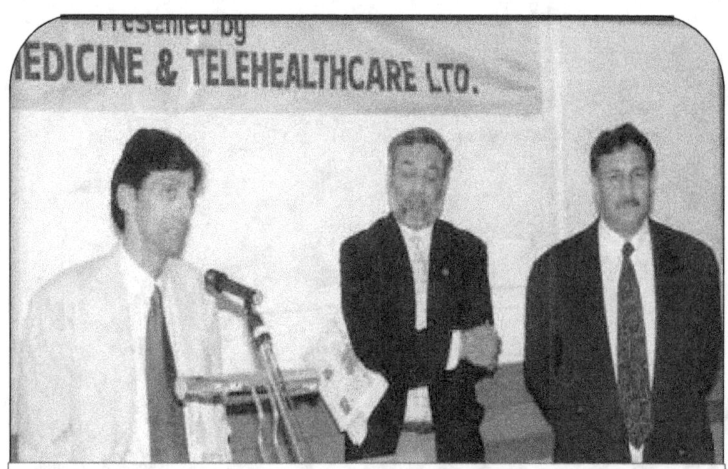

Technology Show presented by Techno Telemedicine & Telehealth Care Ltd. at The Bristol. **Mr. Ashok Sharma of UNESCO** addressing the audience and inviting TTTCL in UNESCO project

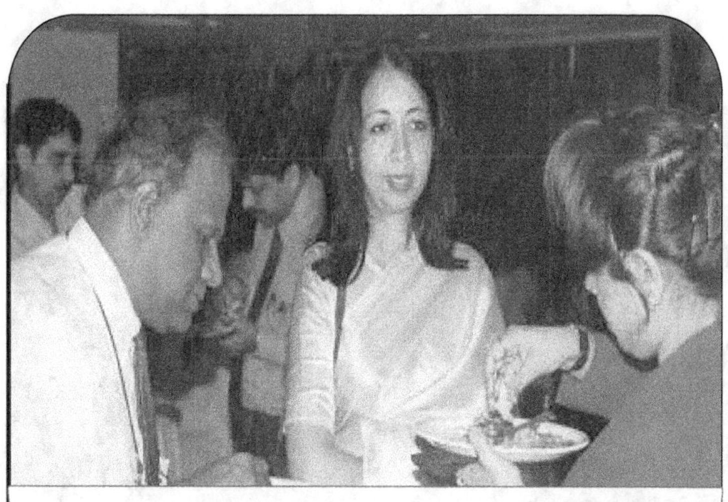

Dr. Abey Koon of WHO during one of our presentations

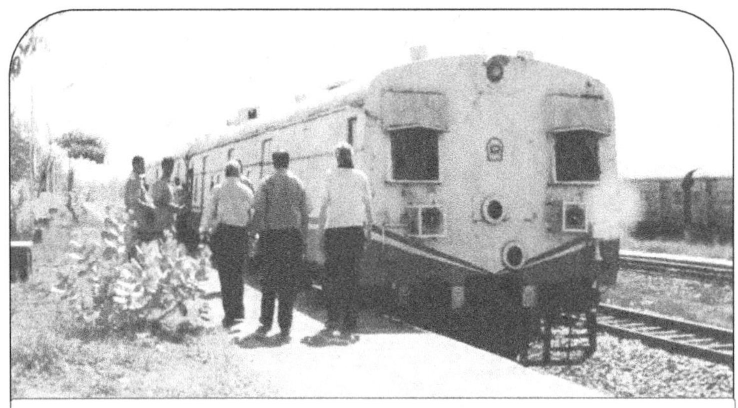

Team Visit
Inspecting the Rail wagons offered by
the Konkan Railways for setting up mobile digital medical center
for show casing technology all over India

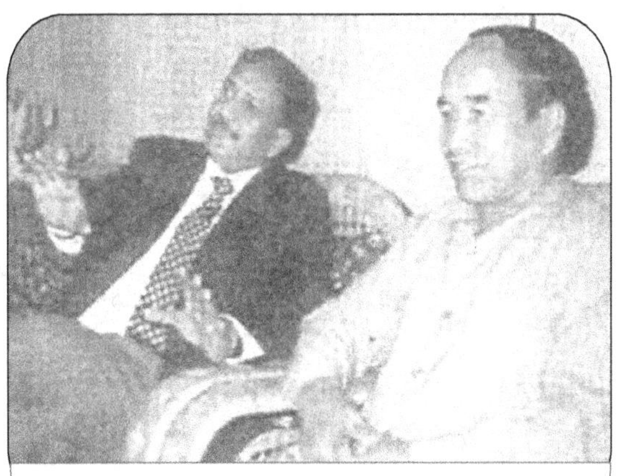

Zoram Thanga , Chief Minister of Mizoram at his
residence at Aizwal with Dr. Arvind Aggarwal

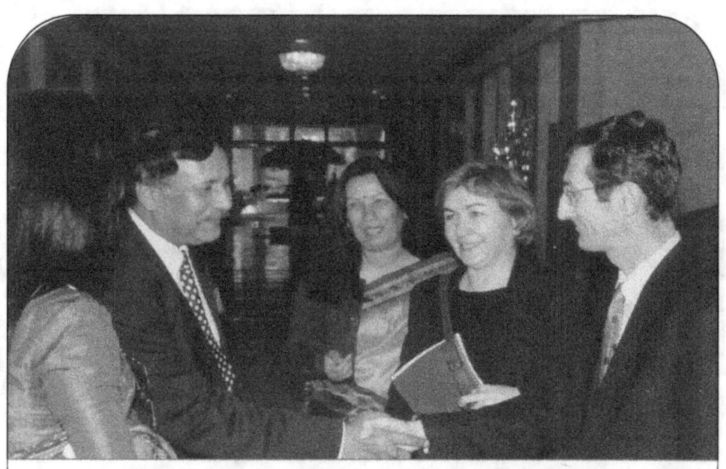

Commendations pour in for the Project Idea of seminal impact

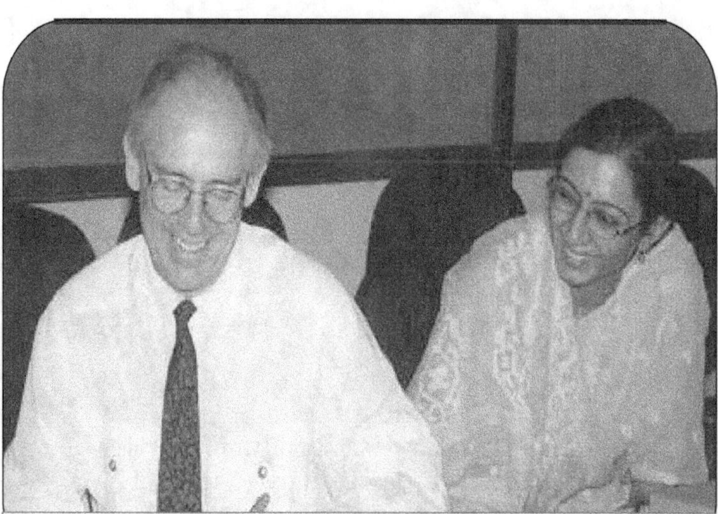

Mr. Mark Sphor of the **US Selection Team for Healthcare in Asia:
New Technologies - New Options**
during a discussion with Dr. Aggarwal

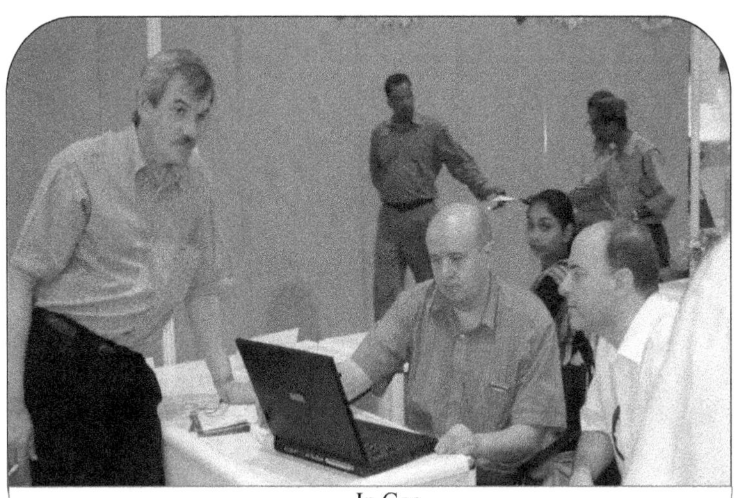

In Goa.
Standing: Robert Phillips. Working at the laptop: Dag
Christensen from Rikshospitalet & Bjorn from Telenor

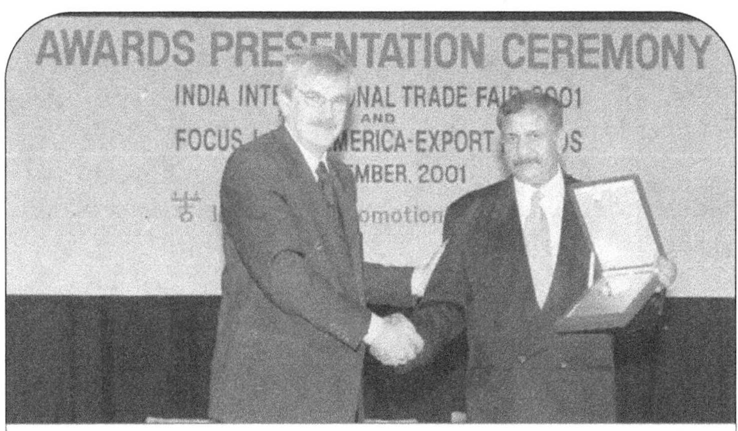

National and Global Awards
In recognition of the Vision of Universal Healthcare

Chapter 15

THE BEGINNING

Unfortunately, the project could not be executed for want of adequate advancement in technology. But fortunately, we were not ready to roll back. Yet.

My resolve was constant. I WOULD wait it out - as the years rolled by, as technology grew and the world shrunk into that little space that begins with *www.*

* * *

Kashmir Calling!

In 2000, Mrs. Pramila Singh joined me to help take forward the project communication. Once, she arranged an appointment for project presentation with the Chief Minister of Jammu and Kashmir (a state in north India),

Dr. Farooq Abdullah at the J&K House in New Delhi. As luck would have it, I happened to be under weather with a sprained ankle, so the team just went ahead to visit the CM on the appointed day.

We had a ready demo kit that contained a laptop, a projector with a screen for showing the video presentation. The 12 minutes of the presentation revealed the full scope of a spectacular mission, laying out its objectives, the implementation mechanism and its monumental impact towards saving lives.

After watching the full length of the video, Dr. Abdullah asked Pramila, "Who is this man who could build this wonderful project?"

When she told him about me, he asked, "Why did he not come?"

She replied simply, "He is not well."

Dr. Farooq Abdullah then said, "No, you are telling a lie . . . He must be a very big man and he purposely could not make the time to come and visit us here."

She repeated politely, "No Sir, he is not well…"

At this, Farooq *Saab* said, "Well, let me speak to him" and asked to connect with me.

"Dr. Aggarwal, I am very deeply impressed with your idea. I have arranged a presentation for the project at the Medical College, Jammu. Will you come? " A man of medicine himself, Dr Farooq Abdullah was genuinely upbeat.

A few days later, the team flew to Jammu to a warm airport reception by the Principal, Medical College of Jammu and senior members of his staff.

The next morning, the whole faculty of Medical College (Jammu), Medical College (Srinagar) and a few others were there to attend the presentation. It was a very long and interesting interaction and we found a lot of young minds particularly enthusiastic about the primary physician's role at the DMCs.

* * *

Let's Go to Goa!

In my journey from *an Idea* to its Imple mentation, I have had the support of many conscientious minds that were dedicated towards upholding public welfare for greater good.

The then Chief Minister of Goa, late Dr. Manohar Parrikar, once met us at the Goa House in New Delhi for a discussion that was preceded by a screening of the Project video.

It was at 7 am the next morning that we were ushered straight into his wood-panelled suite at the guesthouse. He was seated cross-legged, waiting for us. Despite the formal setting, everything about him was informal but matter-of-fact. A man of enterprise with a quick wit, Dr. Parrikar held a Ph.D fr om Indian Institute of Technology (IIT). About half -way into the discussion, he said, "Arvind, I AM SOLD . What do you want? . . ."

"Let's go to Goa. . . We start it from there ," I replied instantly.

Our accommodation and   other logistics were overseen by the Goa Government guesthouse. My full team including daughter Shilpi who'd begun evincing serious interest in the Project, worked through the days to study the landscape and demographics of the state. We returned to the guesthouse only late evenings after spending long days working at the CM's office as we built and customised an implementation roadmap for Goa.

On submission of our Study Report for Goa, Dr. Parrikar instructed the Health Secretary to release the requisite funds towards implementing the projetc. Interestingly, this gentleman put his foot down, citing bureaucratic hurdles, one of which was that there 'needs to be a minimum of three quotations' so that he could award us the contract out of the competition. And perhaps not entirely unforeseen, the advertisement for quotations could not elicit the required response: there were no other contestants. He was adamant that because there were 'no three quotes', contract could not be awarded . . . so it was aborted there. But before we left, Dr. Parrikar organised a particularly warm farewell for us (replete with dinner and folk dance) in addition to a 'promotion event' of a presentation-meeting at the Medical College, Goa.

* * *

The Mizoram Ravines

At the behest of Mr. Zoram Thanga, the then Chief Minister of Mizoram, we travelled to Mizoram as his official guests. Our presentation was attended by a full house of the State Assembly members including the Chief Minister and all min isters of Cabinet rank.

Mr. Thanga, at the end of that presentation, regaled us with his recollections of how he'd remained, for very many days, in the ravines of Mizoram, as a rebel. While the connection of his story to the project wasn't immediately apparent, we were issued a letter of intent that once any Indian state has one operating centre, they shall undertake to implement the project all over Mizoram, signed under his name.

It became clear only later that through his stories, Mr. Thanga was perhaps iterating his recognition of a Revolution.

***

Do-er's Delhi!

Dr. A.R. Antuley was the Union Health Minister when Pramila arranged fo r an appointment for our presentation at the Secretariat in New Delhi.

In addition to the senior members of his staff including the Director General of Health Services (Dr. Mukherjee), Dr. Antuley gave us a full hearing. (Indeed the appointment was supposed to be for a duration of 10 minutes but he did not leave for a good two hours). During this time, there was a volley of questions from all quarters and it seemed to me that **the Idea** was steadily gaining ground as I explained the finer nuances of the project, hopefully converting non-believers into committed collaborators. It seemed a very constructive exercise largely because of the range of queries on the points of convergence of Medical Science and Information Technology.

But I especially remember the encounter with this one person who seemed to constantly intercept the flow of discussion, so much that at one point Dr. Antuley rose from his seat in the front row, asked for the mike and remarked, "I am not a Doctor of Medicine, but I sure am a 'Doctor' of common sense... And I can plainly see the difference between a do-er and an auditor!"

* * *

Mission Russia

In 2017, I had an opportunity to visit Russia along with a trade delegation of CII. They'd organised visits to some very interesting tech-based venues in the main cities.

I found Moscow, in particular, dotted with a very large number of what were called *Technology Parks*, where diverse Tech companies operate, conducting research and showcasing their work in relation to the recent technological advancements. I also found that these companies were funded by the government which sees to it that they enjoy the best facilities that help keep their country at the top of the technological game.

Typically for all of Russia, most of the technology is devoted towards actively developing techniques and tactics that are useful in the airspace such as arms and aerial drones.

I was especially astonished to find that one of the Tech companies manufactured batteries that had the power to fly aeroplanes. On the lines of electrical vehicles such cars (or the e-rickshaws in India), aeroplanes could now fly without fuel!

My interest was further piqued to see this company offer us drones that could be customised to deliver medicines, blood and even act as (drone) ambulances. This could really help take the 'Remote Healthcare' concept to the next level. Besides, Russia has a super huge geographical area and in contrast, a very sparse population. Add to it, the harsh weather conditions that prohibit mobility, and Russia could be seen as a really big potential market for the project.

* * *

After Moscow, we flew to Tatarstan (capital Kazan).On reaching the hotel, I was warmly received by Maria, a cheerful young girl who'd kindly agreed to help me as a private interpreter in my appointment with the Health Minister, Tatarstan.

In fact, we left for the meeting right away, as the appointment was allotted for the time right after my plane landed.

On the way, Maria and I chatted about her family and I told her about my mission. She said that she was from Siberia. Her mother still lived there. And that she was here to try and earn a livelihood for both her Mum and herself. Her father had died a year ago after taking seriously ill and not being able to access medical help. Maria was touched to hear about *the Idea*. She keenly listened to the details of the project and said that while she had never heard anything like this, she was certain that it could really help save a lot of lives once it 'comes up' in her country.

At the Minister's office, going through the security protocols took almost an hour, delaying us further. When we reached the Minister's chambers, his Secretary informed us that he was very busy and with great difficulty, we had been granted a 15 minutes' time to explain our "programme" to him.

After thanking the Secretary very politelyfor her help, we stepped into the Health Minister's cabin. It was a warmly lit rectangular room that featured one central marble countertop table where the Minister was seated, extending out into an elaborate seating area for visitors and members of the staff.

By the time we left his chamber, it was 10 pm - we'd spent nearly two hours with him. His Secretary just about managed to stifle a big yawn as she saw us emerge from his chamber. As we bid her *Good night* she remarked, "He never has such a long meeting. This is exceptional!" Am not entirely sure whether she was just making a statement or that was a complaint.

But the Health Minister was fascinated. He'd mindfully heard the presentation, examined the project papers and finally going all out in his commendation, declared that he was happy to '*Give it a Go!*.' But he needed to see the project in operation, at least a single working DMC anywhere in the world and he would fly to India and award us an international contract for implementing the Project throughout Tatarstan. I remember how the young Maria put her palms together and spontaneously clapped in appreciation and gratefulness. I could only smile.

Now, it was upto me to get started with the first DMC, *anywhere in the world*

* * *

Uttar Pradesh Makes the Cut!

2017. The Government of Uttar Pradesh (a State in North India) organised a widely publicised Investors' Summit in Lucknow.

We attended the presentations made by the Minister of Industries, Mr. Sachin Mahana and the Additional Chief Secretary and Commissi oner of Industry, Mr. Anup Chand Pandey. Sure enough, Monica Seth (our Project team member) went and asked the Commissioner of Industries for a meeting. She stated, matter-of-factly,

"We would like to show you a presentation on Digital Medical Centre."

Nonplussed, he asked, *"What is a DIGITAL MEDICAL CENTRE?"*

She smiled slightly and said,"We will show you." He flipped open his wallet to give her a card with his contact details and asked us to send in an email with a formal meeting request. We got an appointment for the next day. At the end of our presentation, the Commissioner said, *"It's an excellent Project . . . I want to do it in Uttar Pradesh! "*

He called the Secretary, Industry and expressed his desire to sign a Memorandum of Understanding (MOU) with us to "bring this Project to the common citizen of Uttar Pradesh". After 15 minutes, we had made and signed the MOU.

* * *

The Land of the Universal (Healthcare) Sun!

By now, Dag (Christensen) was after me to go ahead with the implementation of the Project. After a gap of nearly 17 years, I was not too sure if we were still ahead of time. But before taking the leap to take the Project to foreign shores, I wanted to test the waters.

Around 2018, we were planning to visit Japan for a family vacation. I wrote a paper and submitted it to a forthcoming conference to be organised by the World Academy of Science, Engineering and Technology in Tokyo, Japan. I was surprised when they accepted it. To know that my *Idea* of *Universalisation of Healthcare* to the last nook and cranny of the world was still acceptable at the end of 2 decades, was a relief!

We planned our Japan trip in a way that we could spare at least a day for me to attend the Tokyo Conference (19th International Conference on Health Informatics and Tele-Medicine-2017) and present my paper.

The day before the conference, I took the train from Osaka so I could reach Tokyo by afternoon and check into a hotel well in time for the conference the next morning. But a combination of different factors, including my managing to lose my way, delayed my arrival at the conference venue. By the time I reached, my turn had been passed up.

Fortunately, the organisers, very kindly, agreed to accept me as the last presenter of the session. I started by presenting my Mission, through my paper titled '*IT-*

based Global Healthcare Delivery System: An Alternative Global Healthcare Delivery System'- explaining my vision for a healthy and happy world in the twenty first century, a world that was truly on the go. My words formed of themselves in the packed auditorium that evening. As I spoke, I could see the Project unfolding through my mind's eye. The DMCs spread across cities and small villages in remote areas, patients being attended to by Doctors and Consultants of different nationalities, medicines being delivered at the patient's doorstep. A universal coverage made possible through digital aid and united resolve. And I could feel at that moment, the audience joining me in feelin g the same. As I concluded, I was broken out of my reverie by the audience rising to its feet amidst thunderous applause.

Almost at the same time, I noticed that I was getting calls from my daughter and wife who had no idea of the delay in my presentation time and were anxious about where I was. I bid a hasty 'Goodbye' and rushed out of the venue to go to the railway station to catch the train back to Osaka.

Back home after a few days of the Japan visit, I received the certificate for " *Best Presentation Award for Outstanding Work"* from the World Academy of Science Engineering and Technology, Japan.

I guessed I was still in time for the Project.

Chapter 16

FROM IDEA TO IMPLEMENTATION

With the advent of the latest technology, I began to ponder over what could be the best way to transform the *Vision* into reality. I began to study the technology closely and realised that internet-based applications (commonly known as 'Apps') that are mobile-compatible have permeated our lives as we live it today in a fundamental way. A *Facebook* or a *WhatsApp* or an *Amazon* were great cases in point.

Given their relevance and utility, such apps demonstrate massive growth in popularity across geographies and cultures. It seemed to become increasingly evident to me that an internet-based project that enabled physical devices to wirelessly connect over the internet would be the way forward to surpass the restrictions of space, time and geography. And thus, we can reach out. **To EVERYONE. EVERYWHERE.**

ANYTIME.

Therefore, my ideation of a Universal Healthcare project was likely to benefit from this modality of app-based identity and operation that does not suffer territorial or time-zone limitations.

I started work at putting together the blueprint for project implementation.

I was burning the proverbial midnight oil and everything was going fine until I faced a roadblock. How do we integrate the multifarious diagnostic devices to the app, so that we could achieve instant test results and zero 'wait-time' lapse?

I put the question to my technical team and together we brainstormed for many weeks until we succeeded in finding just the right digital devices that were "integratable" yet low cost.

We customised our own Tele-Medicine console to provide the optimal solution (the MVP Plan) to seamlessly integrate most of the devices that are used in the healthcare industry around the world.

In the process, we ended up with a **Universal Healthcare App** that is packed with user-friendly features as well as the maximum number of clinical diagnostic devices, marking a definite improvement over all other Tele-Medicine consoles that existed erstwhile. The App uniquely advances the system to integrate all commonly-used medical devices such as digital multipurpose camera, digital stethoscope, digital thermometer and other digital equipments that gauge blood pressure, respiration rate, pulse, ECG, besides all blood investigations like Hb, TLC, DLC, Sugar and Kidney function tests, Liver function tests, Lipid profile, and all imaging devices such as X-ray, Ultrasound, CT scan and CT Angiography.

Thus, the App brings home a one-stop digital

healthcare solution. One that was long overdue. Encompassing practically every device used in healthcare industry, but standardising them to meet the most rigorous international quality mandates, this App ensures healthcare at its best.

We worked at developing the App to its best version, running it through countless trials and re-trials until we froze upon its structure.

The Front end is Android and iOS based. Here, the patient may choose to fix the Doctor's appointment at the Digital Medical Centre (DMC) or avail the 'Doctor-at-home' (Visit) option. All beneficiaries such as Doctors, Consultants, Hospitals, Pharmacies, and Laboratories register themselves and confirm appointments/transactions here. This also includes facilitation by ot her app-based partner organisations such as Ola/Uber (to organise the seamless and speedy transportation of Doctors/Consultants and/or patients) and any other(s). The *Front-end* Patient Management system also incorporates a secure provision for online payment for the services.

The Mid web-based portion integrates all digital medical devices, video conferencing software, cloud-based EMR [15]which saves patient information in voice, text, images and video; all of it in encrypted format to be retrieved on-demand. Patient EMR – that integrates all digital medical devices commonly used for examination such as stethoscope, ECG, vital sign monitor, general medical examination camera, X-ray, MRI, CT SCAN, ultrasound, lab investigation devices for routine and special investigat ion of blood and urine and the software shall incl ude facilitation for:

- Speech to text
- Instant multi-lingual translation software
- Chatbot (*WhatsApp*), live chatand

• Video conferencing software

Cloud-based EMR where patient information is captured in audio -visual-text and video format with complete cyber security (encrypted end-to-end) .[16]

The ***Back-end*** handles the E-commerce integration towards receiving /splitting and distribution of all payments received from patient(s) and disbursal amongst all service providers, partners and beneficiaries. All such payments, receipts, splitting and transfers/ reimbursements auto-conduct as per tagged instructions. The App incorporates a multiple-currency feature to seamlessly handle receipts, splitting, conversions and part-conversions as well as reimbursements across geographies. Besides, it contains the multilingual software capability for instant transaction of text and speech.

There is also a 'Knowledge' module containing the various educational and training videos for all device models,[17] rendering it a complete and comprehensive **end-to-end IT-based Universal Healthcare delivery system** . The App also offers an interface for integration of the Hospital Manager Software (HMS) to capture full patient information such as the various investigation reports and/or surgical and/or invasive/non-invasive procedure details along with audio-visual, text and/or video in the available formats. Besides, the App offers a dedicated financial and insurance interface. Artificial Intelligence (AI) and Machine Learning (ML) play a particularly strong role in this IT-based global healthcare delivery system. For instance, should one need to retrieve a particular patient file with 100% accuracy, 100 times, without any mistake, in a split second; it may be a tough call to develop the human competency required to achieve this, and even then, it cannot be ensured that such human intervention will be absolutely perfect each time.

This system preserves images and all other information in chronological order. As a result, auditing information for medico-legal purposes and for assessment of progress or deterioration becomes easy.

Storage of data in the form of images, videos and text includes a particular sequence of date, day and time-wise allocation to standardise and pace up the retrieval process. Hence, the retrieval process in a different sequence like ECG with Arrhythmia needs the specialised software with built-in AI/ML. As a result, the 'intelligent' system can read images and advise best options in diagnosis whether it's ECG, Pathology slides, X-ray, Ultrasounds or Angiography.

Rome was not built in a day. We started with MVP while adding new modules based on availability and demand as we went forward. And Oh! the thrill of building the road as we move ahead onto uncharted territories!

This system is stable, bug-free and 100% robust. I promise. What this system also helps to do is achieve *Objectivity* and *Transparency* in the process. Today, in many ways, we must rely entirely on patients' feedback for assessment.

Such subjective assessment entails the patient declaring whether s/he is feeling better, ie. is the pain or fever any better or worse. In contrast, the *objectivity* in-built in the system ensures that the physician can refer and/or compare the images for assessment of the wound condition. Besides, the system makes it plausible that a number of professionals can simultaneously give medico-legal or clinical opini on at the same or different time(s). This system elimina tes human errors to the maximum extent and renders evaluation transparent and objective.

***

A 'Made in *(Digital)* India' Solution

The first thing I do as I wake up in the morning is check my *WhatsApp*. And this has been my practice over the last couple of years or so. Yet, even 10 years ago, we had no clue how profoundly an app will change the way we communicate and reach out to friends and family. Freeing the world of the cobwebs of STDs and ISDs, *WhatsApp* revolutionised the world of communication quite radically to render communication free (powered through internet), universal and on-the-go. In the world of healthcare, for far too long and for far too much, people have suffered, ached and put up with monstrous pain and distre ss while 'in-waiting'.

It's sure time things changed for the better. It's sure time the delivery of healthcare was freed of the age-old ramshackle of wealth, influence and proximity. That healthcare was made universal, diagnosis was made autonomous and the treatment process truly democratic by choice of access. We, in India, have found the way to do this. Through an app that will revolutionise the delivery of healthcare to people the world over.

Introducing

Sevati (Universal Healthcare) App

After our work spanning 3 decades (starting in 1993 with a simple brainwave), we've finally built a system that reaches healthcare to the remotest corner of the world. Connecting every man, woman and child to a state-of-the art Digital Medical Centre that operates as a physical health booth and that can also travel home to the patient. In the dead of the night or middle of the day. Bringing to the patient a global hub of consultants, physicians, hospitals and even pharmacists. And most importantly, freedom from *wait time,* powered by an automated 27/7 digital infrastructure that also incorporates digital investigations and instant test results such that treatment can start at once. Thus ensuring universalisation of healthcare delivery in its truest, finest and fastest form.

Yet, rewind 2 decades - and this vision would seem unreal. The concept had to be shelved repeatedly for lack of technological advancement. Just like accessing the most inaccessible and remote area to conduct a medical camp, I feel, at those junctures, we were guided by the mind's compass to ensure:
- Upgraded world-class healthcare
- At minimal cost to patient
- Ensuring instan t accessibility.

Getting adequate technical support is key to the implementation of this project. And even back in the day, when Dr. V S Ramamurthy (the then Secretary, Ministry of Science and Technology) and I discussed this with data scientists from ISRO, they used to suggest transponders and satellites to get that kind of bandwidth. Costing upto several lacs of rupees at the time, VSAT, too, offered only a small bandwidth, expressed in kbps. Today, a content creator in the remotest village self-shoots videos and uploads them on the internet for worldwide broadcast instantly. The unit of data measure, 'Kbps' is perhaps not even heard now. Even to me, it sounds like an antique thing, long blown away with the sands of time. Today we can finally implement something we could not do in 2000 because of tech limitations.

And this through a uniquely *Made in (Digital) India* solution: **the Sevati (Universal Healthcare) App** which has created a self-managed and self-financed world-class Universal Heal thcare delivery model.

* * *

INDIA SHINING into a Healthy Future

Can India lead the global implementation of a *Universal Healthcare System* and emerge as the Healthcare capital of the World?

Let's find out.

Digital devices used in the system shall be able to deliver instant reports at virtually no cost to the patient.

The cost of equipment is so low that over time, instead of referring patients for investigations at third-party agencies, every doctor would like to set up a low-cost in-house lab fo r instant investigation at a low cost.

Besides, every clinic will, over a period of time, upgrade to a self-sufficient state-of-art Health Mall, having its own diagnostic laboratory and connected globally to every brand of hospital. Just like a shopping mall hosts multiple brands, every Clinic shall function as a multi-Hospital Clinic. And patients shall have the autonomy to choose from a huge assortment of hospitals or consultants at low cost, a far cry from the long hours spent in the *waiting rooms* of clinics and hospitals. For the first time, Quality Healthcare will be accessible to every person irrespective of geography and socio-economic status.

The Digital Medical Centres will direct the supply of medicines and blood to areas with zero or low road connectivity through drones.

Emergency can be notified and critical patients from far-flung areas such as a remote Siberian village or an inaccessibly steep hill in Nepal or the Himachal, can be transported through drones to DMCs and hospitals. While the patient is being transported to the hospital, pre-arrival emergency arrangements can be made towards

- Arranging blood
- Arranging surgical team and
- Preparing operation theatre.

NO MATTER WHERE, NO MATTER WHEN,

be it earthquake-hit zones or war-torn areas or flooded regions, be it airplanes or ships   , **LIVES CAN BE SAVED** .

Yet, the next phase of innovation in the system will make it possible that even the most critical operations can be performed in a remote area under the guidance of consultants, and without the patient having to be moved over a distance. This phase of the project envisages the DMCs be extended as **Robotics Surgery Centres.**

Wasn't it roughly 3 decades ago when we would write letters to loved ones in hand ? A time when it would sure have been fanciful to imagine a day in the near future when letter-writing would be a digital, fast-paced and instant process. And yet, here we are!

Compare this phenomenon with robotic surgery, which is already catching on. In conventional letter-writing, we used to write a letter by hand (not type). Compare it with the conventional mode of surgery done by hand. Every single surgery is different just as each time we write, every hand-written word is different. Only here, there are lives at stake - and a single microscopic miscalculation can cost us dearly.

Returning to the writing analogy, next came 'type'. Where the font was standardised, all gaps and page settings were standardised. However, once typed, mistakes could not be edited.

Until, finally we arrived at electronic writing through computer keyboards and of course, texting through mobile phones. Writing (especially with swipe facility), now is faster, neater and amenable to swift corrections.

This is exactly how surgery for critical ailments or organ transplants will benefit through robotic procedures. Surgery at the robotic DMC is faster, neater and most importantly, accurate -ie there is least bleeding, least about for complications and minimal recovery time, with the patient getting back on his/her feet faster. This means that now we have a computer interface (which has taken tens of thousands of hours' work to get to this point of perceptive software precision) guiding these imprecise human hands of ours. Thus, the precision of scale comes into the picture and suddenly we gain complete control. Transitioning to this system is our safest bet to a scenario where we have 100% success rates in surgeries.

There are, sadly, enough reported accidents of a small instrument such as a gauge having been left inside the patient body during surgery. Sometimes, there are more shocking incidents. An incident as recent as November 2022 comes to mind where the news media reported the unfortunate occurrence of a critical body organ being stolen. We will perhaps not be able to instantly rid the world of its many ills, but we will, for sure, ensure that the frequency of their occurrence is on a fast decline. Technology-based surgeries, video recording of procedures and other modes go a long way in standardising and thereby preventing mishaps of any nature or kind.

Which brings us to the magic of **Standardisation** , an innovation that the Universal Healthcare App incorporates. With the advent of technology, standardisation through high-quality devices and processes can bring about a hitherto untapped resource base that strea mlines and secures the quality of the processes being leve raged across board.

Given that every institution has a different design and a different architecture, research shows that standardising designs renders work practical and productive.

For instance, say, you are about to board a train for your journey. You know exactly how many berths will be there in your compartment, and which one amongst them is yours. You will know where the washrooms are located and what is their design.

The same can be replicated for every industry that deals with services essential to life and health. Standardised designs help create economy of scale, such that things can be made better, cheaper and easier toinstall, main tain and use.

The Universal Healthcare system tries to achieve optimal standardisat ion of procedures, equipments and designs.

A Standardisation of
- **Design**
- **Equipments**
- **Procedures**
- **Educational/Training material**
- **Pricing and**
- **Services**, helps brings standardised world-class healthcare to the world, like one global currency.

However, standardisation of services is a challenge given the variable human factor. To address this, the smart digital system incorporates various training modules that are educational videos (also available through links) that can be an inexpensive and easy mode of knowledge-sharing for the doctors. These pre-recorded lecture modules, say, on how to use a digital device, impart both theoretical and practical knowledge in a standardised way to begin with.

Besides, through standard process and equipment learning, even surgical procedures and clinical interventions may be accessible to physicians based on the case requirements.

Moreover, the doctors, especially at the DMCs, working under the guidance of global consultants, will naturally undergo continuous medical and surgical education, raising the bar for competency and experience.

Visualising such a comprehensive system of Healthcare delivery is perhaps not too formidable if we can, for a moment, return to the example of   *WhatsApp*.

Ten years ago, a telephone call was audio-based, costly (remember those pages of postpaid bills!) and poor quality (poor network, fre quent cross connections!).

Today: *WhatsApp call is*

• *Audio - visual,*
• *High quality, and*
• *Free globally.*

Thinking of these lines, we're at the brink of redefining Healthcare delivery through the **Sevati App,** that ensures:

World class Healthcare
Instantly
For Everyone
Everywhere
Anytime
At lowest cost (substantively free).

The Mission is to bring world-class global healthcare to everyone. After long years (that have slipped into decades) of conceptualising an idea from its vague rudimentary form to developing it to the sophisticated digital infrastructure it is today, the system is up and running and I dream of the day when the benefits of this system will be hand-del ivered to men and women of nations large and small.

In hindsight, I never thought I'd design a remote digital healthcare system. I just had this compelling continuous thought that there needs to be a system which can treat people even remotely. (A thought which garnered increased acceptability in the post-Covid era). As a young medical student conducting medical camps, especially in Himachal, I closely saw how people in remote villages often could not access a doctor or hospital. Patients often died on the way as terrains were difficult, especially during snowfall or rains when the mud roads would be washed away or at best, rendered inaccessible. Interestingly now, the mobile phone with YouTube has made it to these regions, but the Doctor hasn't.

* * *

The Doctor is Home!

In the seven decades that I've lived, amongst the very many social changes that I've witnessed, particularly interesting has been the slow waning away of the familiar face of the 'Family Doctor'. That iconic figure in old films, who was ready to 'visit' with his black bag whenever called and sit by the bedside wielding his stethoscope. The GP (General Practitioner) who's chamber was conveniently located down the lane, three or four houses away or perhaps on the next street. No matter what the ailment (a splitting headache or a sudden fever, a runny nose or a coughing throat) - he was there to provide instant relief. Primarily because he was the 'Family Physician'. He knew the patient's history of illnesses, symptoms and allergies and could quickly and effectively ameliorate.

So, the GP was the primary point of contact and the gateway to good health, it was he who would 'refer' the patient to the Specialist where needed.

But there are always more people coming in for minor ailments or age-related issues that do not need specialised attention than for major or critical illnesses.

Through this, my life's work, I've tried to build the bridge between the utterly depersonalised approach of an App by incorporating the merits of once again sending the local GP home to the patient (this time as the DMC Doctor). For the soothing words and reassuring touch as much as the quick relief from sudden alarming situations or the periodic management of hypertension, asthma or blood sugar. Thus, sparing the patient both monetary expense and exertion of finding an able companion and the right transportation.

At the stage where the Specialist must be sought, the urban cities and towns are teeming with multi-speciality clinics where the patient must 'go' and await the Specialist's attention, thereafter trailing numerous expensive tests. Even this would have been alright had the record-keeping not been such a scary, if not entirely nerve-racking proposition. Every one of us suffers different problems in the body at different points in time, and often multiple issues simultaneously. So, the patient's 'kidney' ailment file may be in one hospital, and she may have sought another Doctor in the other multi-Speciality for her 'heart' condition, and her 'knees' may yet be on another floor of the same. This situation would had been positively funny, if it were not so unwieldy and taxing for the patient or the carers to track and explain the full case history of ailments, fishing out the X-rays, ECGs, prescriptions and medicines that were advised and taken each time.

The **Sevati Universal Healthcare** App is a tap away. It is on the phone screen of the elderly parent whose children live many many miles away. Or the farm help who lives far away from the nearest super-speciality hospital. Or just about anyone who wishes to autonomously seek effective healthcare. It is technology at its best. And its noblest.

Loss of time has plagued healthcare for far too long. It's perhaps about time, we kissed it one final *Goodbye!*. This, my life's work, is for you.

FRIENDS AND FAMILY

Dr. Meena Aggarwal

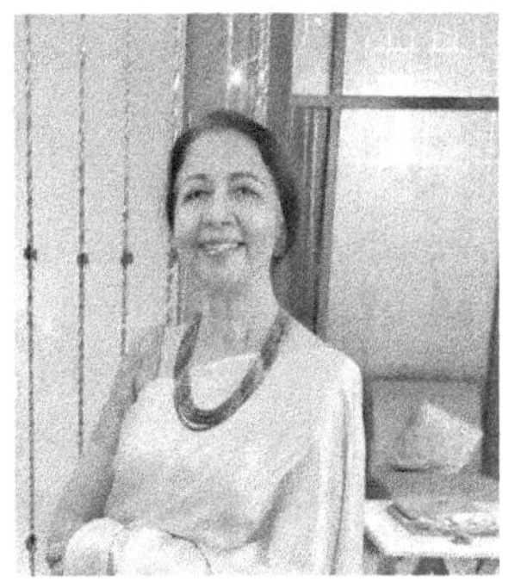

"   My grandfather was an Arya Samaj reformist while my father was an atheit. it don't remember ever having visited a temple as a young child or even praying at home. On the other hand, Arvind had been brought up to believe in Sanatana dharma (Hinduism). In the early days after our marriage, we used to go for morning walks. On the way, there was a temple. Arvind usually went in to pay his homage. However, just before going in, he would ask, "Would you like to come in?" I would shake my head in the negative and wait outside the temple for him. This continued for days together. But never even once did he insist that I come inside or do a *puja* (prayer). He respected my freedom to choose. It was much later that I began to go in and sit down to wait for him rather than stand outside the premises. Eventually, of course, I discovered for myself, the joy of doing a *puja*

Arvind is a workaholic. He enjoys his work and always tries to do his best. No matter how big or difficult the task may be, he will give his all to accomplish it. He is a firm believer in "Quitters never Win & Winners never Quit". It is perhaps this mindset that has kept him going at the Tele-Healthcare projec these last 3 decades and counting!

He believes in making it large (*pun intended*). *"You have to work for the same number of hours . . . And in that time, you could either do something ordinary and small. Or something big and extraordinary. The time taken is the same, so why do something small?*- is how he explains it. I vividly recollect the time he got an export order for 70,000 dozens of T-shirts back in 1986. We had never made T-shirts and there was an export quota from India. I was very apprehensive but he was certain that he'd find a way. Despite the many hurdles; his grit, perseverance, out-of-the-box thinking and the ability to keep his team together, helped him execute the order successfully through cross-border collaboration! No mean feat this.

With the money that he earned from this order, he bought (again, nothing small!) 20 acres of agricultural land, back in 1988! And he became an example for the whole family - my side and his, for having achieved so much so soon. At 36 years of age and 8 years into the export business, a doctor of medicine had ventured out of his comfort zone, taken some brave and fearless steps and emerged a success story - the kind whose phenomenal life story is stuff that legends are made of!

And along the way, Arvind inspired. As only he can. I remember when Vikash (our son-in-law) was working at the Barclays Bank, Arvind would often jokingly say to him " *Baniye doosron ki naukri nahi karte, apna bank banao!* " (Businessmen don't work for others, make your own bank!)". And I would respond by saying, "*Hey! Isn't that too much to expect?* " But Arvind was sure that it was possible.

There had once been an opportunity, as suggested by his Chartered Accountant, to buy majority of shares in the Bank of Madurai, back in 1988-89, but he wasn't sure as it was a huge amount and he had no experience whatsoever in the field. I guess he pushed Vikash because he'd had to pass up that opportunity.

And then, one day, Vikash announced that they had, in fact, got the licence for a Bank in London - Arvind was beyond the moon! „

Shilpi Gupta (Aggarwal)

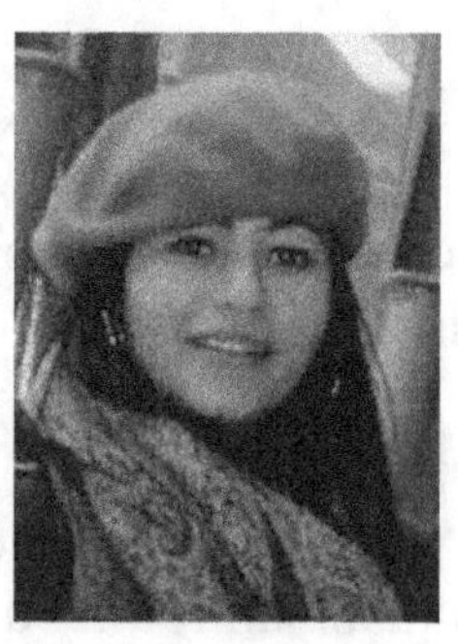

" Dad and I share a lot of common interests, right from our love for *jalebis* (a quintessential Indian dessert comprising crispy yellow spirals filled with sugar syrup) to a unique habit that I picked up from him - before starting out every morning, Dad religiously 'plans' his day - jotting down a list of all the important tasks with a pen in his diary (a constant companion). Some days, I would assist him in making the list and it was just so much fun! Today, my days don't get started without my list of "To Do's".

Dad set the highest goals not just for himself but for everyone around him. I remember that as a young girl just starting college, I'd begun to get interested in fitness. And Dad got me a gym membership at The Radisson, Gurgaon! He insisted that I train at the best of gyms and not the usual ones which dotted our locality. In hindsight, it really made a difference to me as a person as it changed my outlook. Now that I was going to a 5-star gym, I was more aware of my surroundings, how I carried myself, my hair, my posture, indeed all of it. More than anything else, the boost to my confidence was immense.

Dad has exemplary determination. Once he fell ill and was advised by the doctor to quit smoking. For someone who smoked a couple of packets everyday, quitting instantaneously was unimaginable and yet he did it. Just like that! That left a mark in my head of what sheer willpower can achieve!

Another time that revealed his super strong resolve was perhaps one of the most stressful times of our lives when Dad suffered the stroke. Not one but multiple ones while he was at the hospital! His speech was affected with a severe slur and so was his movement - he was unable to walk on his own. But he retained his rock solid determination to return to normal life.

Despite being physically very weak, he began by slowly and painfully walking the lengths of the hospital corridors. Once he returned home, he started a rigorous exercise regimen at the gym. And the incredible results are here. He is strong and sturdy as if nothing ever happened!

In fact, he's quite a riot around his 8-years old granddaughter, Zara. Each time we're back home, Zara and he will wake up to lots of hugs, solve the daily crossword or play UNO, amongst tons of other things! I remember as a baby, Zara was colic child and every night, around 2 am, she would wake up with tummy aches and break into a series of intense painful cries. Dad couldn't bear to see her in pain. I recall the time that he ventured out in the dead of the night to find pharmacies that were open and got her a range of tummy-soothing medicines. Though Zara would refuse to consume any of these, and they weren't really much help, it's his even getting up at that unearthly hour to find her some help, that has stayed on. Only family can do this for you.

I love you, Dad. To the Moon and back! "

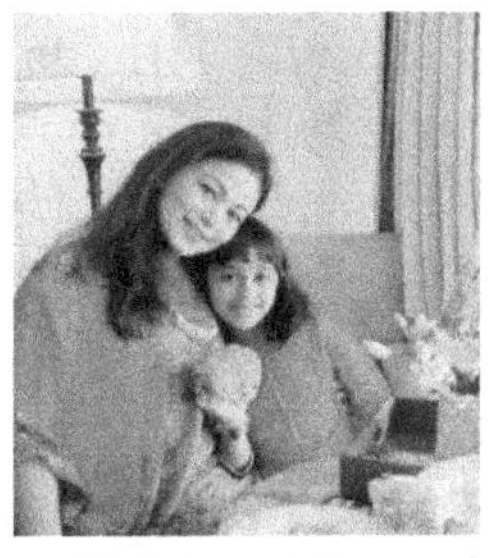

Shilpi and Zara

Vikash Gupta
Co - Founder & CEO of
VAR CAPITAL,
(An Investment
Management company) &
Co - Founder &Non-
Executive Director,
MONUMENT
BANK,London, United
Kingdom

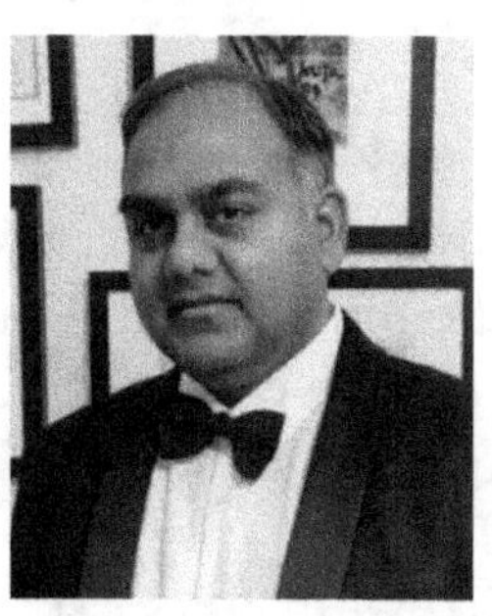

"

While I was
dating Shilpi (my wife)
more than 2 decadesago, I
met Dad at The Bristol (a
5-star hotel in Gurgaon,
India). He was addressing
the press-meet over the
Tele-Medicine Project. I
hadn't been to many press
conferences before this,
and I remember being
super impressed and really
inspired! Dad was way
ahead of his time and he
spoke with awe-inspiring
conviction. Till date, I
continue to be intrigued by
how dynamic he was and
continues to be.

He's just so much
more than a Doctor. His
vision is profound and the
scale of his ambition,
magnanimous. While I was
working at Barclays, he'd
often remark, "*Why do you
work in a Bank? Why don't
you own it?*" At that point,
of course, it felt
impossible. But I guess,
somewhere deep down, his
words left a mark. So, 15
years from then, when I,
along with my two friends,
actually started a bank -
MONUMENT, it was
surreal!

The audacity of his
ambition is inspiring, to
say the least. A lot of
people may find his vision
incredulous. Simply
because one is mostly too
afraid to dream.

He's been through
so many ups and downs,
but he continues to remain
super positive all the time.
And that rubs off on you.
He's very inspiring in that

sense - not afraid to dream big, but also with an abiding determination and single-minded focus to make it real.

And yet, Dad's really simple, straight-forward and has a way of instantly putting you at ease. I'd like to add that he's exceptionally kind and very generous. There was this one time when Mishraji, one of our employees, travelled from Dhanbad to Delhi on some errand for my father, and Dad treated him to a sumptuous meal, even sharing a bottle of wine (all because he looked tired!), afterwards dropping him to the railway station. Till date, Mishraji raves about Dad's generosity and how well he was treated and taken care of.

On the date of my writing this, MONUMENT, despite being a brand new private bank, is serving millionaire clients in the UK through digital technology and has secured full regulatory approval, and I can't not say *'Thanks, Dad! You mean the world to me"*

Professor Anand Mishra
MBBS, MD, (Pathology and Microbiology)
Former Principal & Dean, RDJM Medical College, Turki, Muzaffarpur, Bihar, India

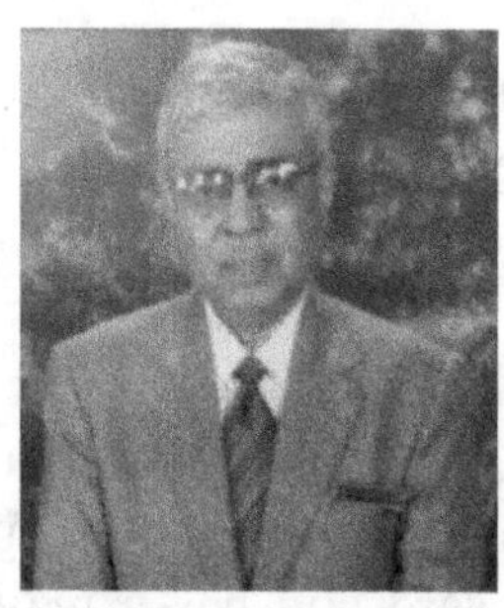

" For as long as I can remember, Arvind had been working on his Dream Project. He developed it over very many years and wherever he presented it, it was highly acclaimed.

But since this was some 3 decades back and IT was not yet developed, it looked futuristic at the time. Now, I feel the time is ripe for this elaborate system of Tele-Healthcare to be launched across the globe. The project implementation is feasible provided it goes into the right hands. Once implemented, it will prove to be a boon for people all over the world. Especially India.

I say, India especially, because the young doctors posted in rural areas are usually absent at their place of work and there may be various reasons for this. But this absence compels the villagers to seek advice from unqualified practitioners (or quacks), leading to mis-diagnosis, incorrect treatment, wastage of money, but most importantly - the loss of time, frequently resulting in irremediable damage.

Seen in this light, Dr. Arvind Aggarwal's Project will be a game changer. Because it is a win-win proposition for the government which can be seen to be providing expert opinion even at the remotest doorstep. The people in general, once they realise how useful, inexpensive and convenient this system is,

will lap it up.
Especially because our memories of the pandemic-induced emergency are still very fresh. During the lockdown, doctors couldn't travel. And patients were unable to approach Doctors even for common ailments. At that time, Tele-medicine, in its most rudimentary form, came to their rescue. We should go into preventive mode before the next crisis strikes and we're again compelled to take desperate measures.

Also, the IT arm of the Project needs to be strong and needs a Murthy or a Nilekani to helm it.

Arvind, through his brainchild, has shown us the way to do it. It's mind-boggling how he got the idea. But what better than for us to gift to the world a *Made in India* solution to the eons-old problem of healthcare delivery and present the *Doctor at the Door*!"

Dr. Ashok Beckaya
Former Paediatrician, the National Health Service, London, United Kingdom

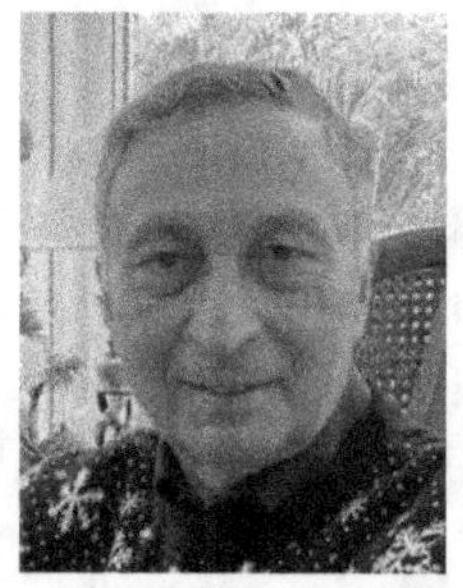

" Arvind and I first met as batchmates at the Medical College, Jamshedpur. In the ensuing years, we largely lost touch.

Communication technology was hardly anything like what it is today. For one, we certainly had no *WhatsApp* to instantly connect!

But once technology broke down the communication barriers, I was back in touch with most of my pals. And with Arvind. He's a special one.

Over the years, Arvind has been dedicatedly working to wards reaching healthcare to every one, irrespective of location and time. I've heard him discuss the work he's doing in Tele-Medicine many many times. So, that's how I realised that he continues to be passionate about it, despite all the years.

I think it's a great *Idea*! From India's perspective, it's just what we've needed for so long. Access to healthcare continues to be a major problem despite the recent improvements in every other sector of human life. The public hospitals have been there since ages, but most failed to ensure accessibility for the masses. So, people who could not reach the big Specialists or Multi-speciality hospitals (mostly located in metropolitan areas), have been largely left to fend for themselves.

Technology has brought about a sea change in the way we do clinical work, especially over the last couple of years. Arvind's Project is based on a seminal idea and a viable technology. And if one looks closely, it's happening in bits and pieces all around the world. And we've all really experienced this during Covid when we were shut out at our homes and we really felt the need to start t h i n k i n g   o f h e a l t h c a r e d e l i v e r y differently than how it was conventionally being done. And we need one Solution t h a t w o r k s a c r o s s populations.

Add to this, the concepts of Effectiveness and Time. One must consider *Whether the patient actually needs to physically visit the Doctor each time?* The fi r s t t i m e - i t's f o r examination. The second visit may be to discuss the investigations. And then the follow-up(s). So, in my line of work (Paediatrics) this means that parents must miss work. And the child, must be taken out of school for at least, the days of 'visit'. Mostly, we find,

that is really unnecessary. So, we look at Arvind's work for the solution. Besides, if you can avoid p a t i e n t s p h y s i c a l l y "walking in" each time, you can avoid exposure for the other patients. That's a lot of goods packed into one.

Yes, Tele-Medicine will change the status quo. And so it will be vociferously resisted. That's bound to happen. But the government needs to c o m e t o A r v i n d andshould agree to take it up through public-private e n g i n e e r i n g . I a m convinced that over time, more support will pour in. From all quarters and segments. So, I really hope we in India, can achieve this for the world. First.

Thanks Arvind! "

Dr. Ashwani Trehan
Gynaecologist
(Endometriosis), London,
United Kingdom

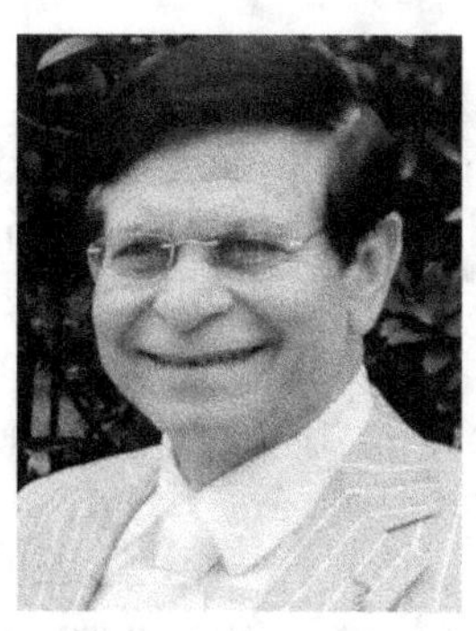

"   Dr. Arvind Aggarwal, I can proudly say, is my friend. Our journey began in 1971 in Jamshedpur where we went to study Medicine at the Mahatma Gandhi Memorial (MGM) Medical College.

Arvind has rare and exceptional achievements in the apparently disparate fields of Medicine and Business. He excelled in the world of Business due to his incredible leadership, vision, dedication, trust, reliability, hard work, creative skills and non-negotiably high standards. There was a demand for his goods not just in India but around the globe.

Despite his phenomenal success in business, Arvind's passion for healthcare and an incessant urge to help humanity contributed to his mission towards creating something exceptional in the world of medicine, too. Arvind showed the way to Tele-Medicine with the aim to bring the hospital home for patients to access timely healthcare and overcome most ailments. With his insight, innovation, professionalism, problem-solving communication, strong ethics and teamwork skills, he took the ethos of Tele-Medicine and Tele-Health to a stage where not only India but also institutions abroad looked at his work with interest and awe, and along the way, came numerous awards and recognitions. Arvind is great example for those who wish to make a positive difference to others' lives through creativity and innovation. I truly admire him and am very proud to be his friend. „

Bob Phillips
Founder CEO
Sustainability Engineering
Centre AS

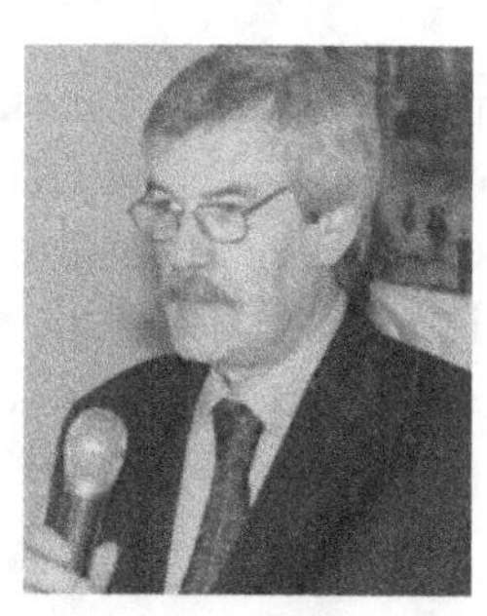

" At the time I met the Doc (Dr. Arvind Aggarwal) and for quite some years earlier, I was at the National Hospital (Norwegian University of Science and Technology), Norway.

It was at this 1999 conference of G8countries (organised by American Telemedicine Service Providers Association and Royal Society of Medicine London) at the Millennium Hotel in London, that I first heard the Doc speak. And what he said left a profound impression on my mind. I was instantly drawn to the strength of his conviction and the nobility of the vision, and we have been buddies ever since.

While I had been working with hearing loss and other specific human disabilities, Dr. Aggarwal's Project addressed the human person as a whole. His approach to Healthcare is quite frankly, like nothing I've seen before. In Tele-Medicine, his approach is very rare, no one else does it the way he envisaged it.

Back in my office from the Millennium Hotel in London, I discussed this with my colleagues from Telenor, SINTEF (a prominent Norwegian IT Foundation) and Rikshospitalet (a part of Oslo University), and we conducted meetings with the Doc who came to Norway for the deliberations. Of course, we had great support from the Intervention Center of the Hospital. These guys were working on remote robotic surgery since earlier, and what they were saying fitted in, very nicely, into the Doc's overall philosophy.

Doc is an absolute genius in General Medicine. He's got an understanding of people and patients, that is rare. There was this one time that a lady walked into his chamber - she was perspiring profusely and quite visibly distraught. The Doc listened to her, holding her hand while he spoke to her, and offered her bananas. It was an extremely hot day, and her electrolytes were really low. The bananas revitalised her instantly. That day I saw, at first hand, his deep knowledge and abiding interest in the human nature.

Doc's model will be useful in many lateral ways. For instance, it makes for great opportunity for the young doctors who can now practice their art, working with Specialists and collaborating with community health workers.

We travelled all over India, showcasing the concept, signing MOUs, receiving letters of interest from as many as 15 Indian states. Tata Infotech and Larsen & Toubro signed up as tech partners on the project. Particularly inspiring was the MOU with the Konkan Railways. Our collaboration with Konkan assigned us a plot on the Madgaon station for developing a Digital Medical Centre (DMC). They even allotted us 3 wagons, converting them into mobile DMCs that could travel fr om village to village for live demo. In fact, they committed to the setting up of such DMCs on all stations across India, once the experiment took off on the Konkan belt. Unfortunately, despite the positive enthusiasm; the Project could not move forward due to lack of adequate technological advancement.

But this is typical not just for India. Friends the world over report similar incidents where the best intentions didn't make it. A case in point would be the Paediatric Cardiology section at Oslo Hospital - patients losing the battle to the lack of timely communication. (Technologically, unlike the early 2000s when one had to depend on Satellite communication for bandwidth and the limited terrestrial coverage, now is absolutely feasible to launch the project globally).

In the early 1990s, the biggest barrier in moving things forward was the lack of political will of leaders bent upon maintaining th e status quo. I remember th is one time when we went to Pune University - the response was so heartwarmingly positive - they came all out in full support, firm in the conviction that the Project model was technologically and medically - Viable. The year was 2004.

It's 2023 now. And I'm ready to join forces with the Doc to forge ahead in order to reinvent healthcare. For us everywhere. Once and for all."

Dag Christensen
Senior Advisor
Telemedicine
Oslo University Hospital
OUS Norway

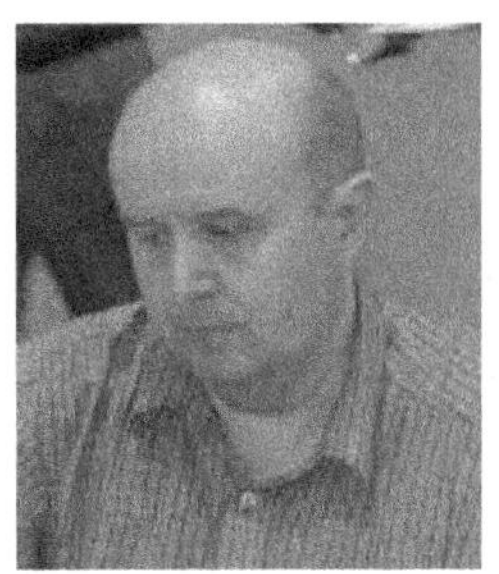

" I first met the Doc (Dr. Aggarwal) during 2000-2001 when we were introduced by Bob (Phillips) in Miami in the United States.

Doc is a man of integrity. He has years of experience and immense practical know-how towards spearheading the Tele-Medicine movement around the world.

I was born in 1958, at a time when remote technology was just about breaking out of its shell. I started out by running a small company in Robotics. People would want a door to appear in the wall, or maybe wish a room to disappear! Or just remove some floors from the building! In fact, we did some very interesting things with boardrooms that could double up as regular office spaces at other times. By the end of the 1980s, I bought my own camera and began to travel with a Doctor. We operated in Copenhagen and could see this at Oslo.

With time, more and more inventions took place in the field of technology. Imagine the patient is on Mount Everest - our job is to see that everything is still in order to support him medically. Tele-Medicine, is practically, army spats: you have instruments in a suitcase that can diagnose anyone, anywhere. Now, that we've 5G, we can literally do this from everywhere.

In a way, Tele-Medicine sees possibilities where there are none. The Doc's idea of Satellite

Medical centres or DMCs is unique. Because for a really long time, we've grappled with how to go about getting it done. For instance, in just about most of our countries, the technology is in place. And funding is mostly sorted, too. But it's the Business model that is the most confoundingly difficult to deal with. With the Doc's Project, there is a solution to that!

Together with the Doc, we've organised a number of presentations and conferences at Oslo University, working closely together in India where I handled the Project booth (at India International Trade Fair). So, it was deeply inspiring. And also, hugely challenging. Of course, I continue to remain very committed to this project as on Day 1.

Sure, there were questions around the feasibility of the idea. What happens when a high-level surgery is planned. Think, a Heart transplant. Or a Lung transplant. Or maybe even Cancer. The Doctor will still operate. Only this time it's that tiny chip that can do it all. Far more accurately too. And that's the Revolution that's waiting to happen. It's on its way. The Doctor's chamber is on your phone. Dr. Aggarwal has offered the optimal solution and we need more force to think and achieve it.

Of course, collaborations would really help such that instead of the one single horse, we can have seven, all pulling in the same direction. Bringing the destination nearer than we thought. There's a lot in it for all of us."

Dr. Ghanshyam Doshi
General Physician and
Philanthropist

" Arvind was always very bright and brilliant. I first met him at the MGM College, Jamshedpur and amongst the very many attractive facets of his personality, the one that struck me the most was Arvind's far-sightedness - it seemed to me that he could see into the future, and that much in advance.

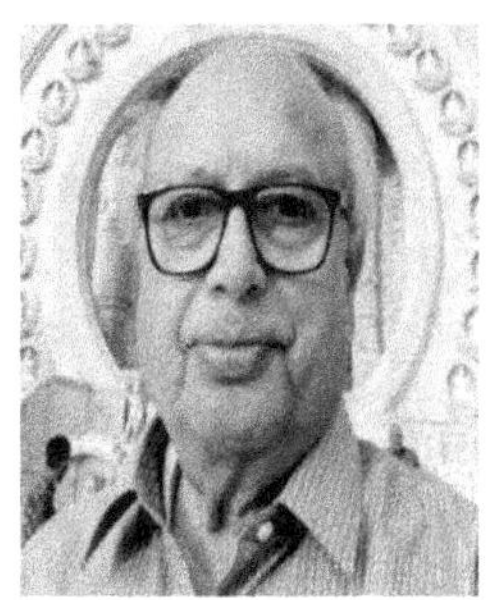

Back in the day in 1995, Arvind visualised setting up Digital Medical Centres that would look into the problem of the lack of accessibility to quality healthcare, especially in the rural areas which have continued to remain geographically cut-off and economically impoverished despite our many years of independence. There will be a structured process for accessing patient data, thereby preempting any time loss. Also, treatment will be much better managed and a lot faster. For the first time, there can be a unified pattern of healthcare delivery at cheaper rates. Technology can be leveraged to bring the fruits of science to everyone. The Project, thus, strongly connects patients, doctors and governments together.

The project's meta-design also helps to generate awareness amongst everyone about the fundamental right to universal healthcare. It is most encouraging that finally we have an app that brings the doctor, the patient, the policymaker and the community worker on the same platform.

We need to convert this exceptional plan to

action immediately. Especially given that Arvind's global healthcare system can be easily leveraged over the internet without the necessity of formidable bandwidths.

I congratulate Arvind on his noble endeavour!"

Ishani Patel
Business Associate & IT
Consultant
Hidden Brains
InfotechPvt. Ltd

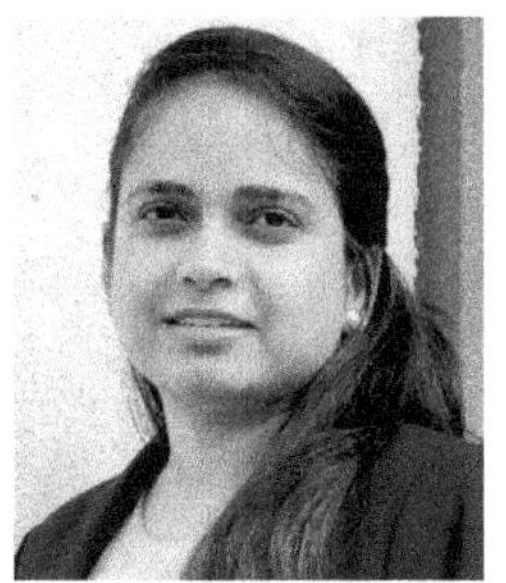

"

As a Business associate, I'm primarily involved in the conceptualisation of the specific requirements and operations to be digitised for the end user. And with Dr. Arvind Aggarwal, the process was as exciting as it gets. For one, he had already worked out an elaborate blueprint to implement the Project vision.

Together with him, we've worked at defining his concept and determining how *the Idea* can be embedded into a software. Given the global magnitude of the application, we looked at multiple options before freezing our solution. The digitalisation of the hospital management system would entail multiple phases starting with the core aspects such as doctors' onboarding, people onboarding, appointments booking, EMR, amongst others.

It will save lives. Especially where fatalities are caused by reasons of medication not reaching the patient on time. Getting connected real time with Specialists is novel and a very empowering tool. Especially in the case of a large population. Now real people can reach out to real people through the project solution. Like never before!

Dr. Aggarwal addresses the healthcare needs of the last person, irrespective of geography, time and clime. Even the one who has no access to technology. Even that person can go to the nearest DMC.

It's a Revolution that I'm sincerely grateful to be a small part of. „

Nadh Thota
Global Technology &
Innovation
(Ex-Wipro, Synaptics,
Wistron, Tata Elxsi, TVS)

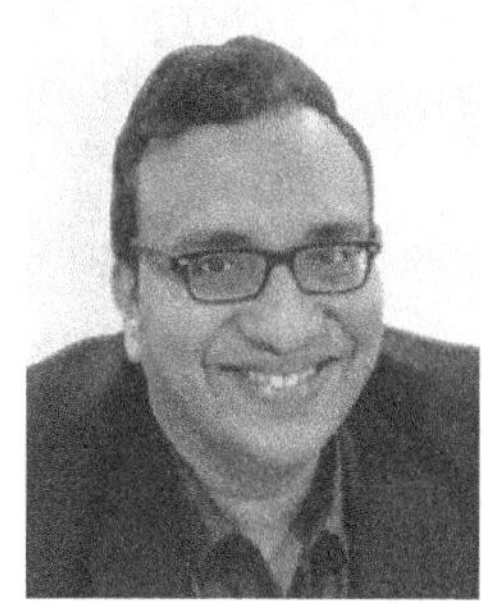

"	I love to say that I *don't* sell commodities. I sell Innovation. I sell the *Future* But never did my words ring more real than when I heard Dr. Arvind Aggarwal relate his ideas of bringing healthcare to the pauper and the prince alike. His process has been vetted time and again by so many experts in healthcare and public policy and he's continued to be passionate and zealous about it over the years.

I think it's a great opportunity for the country to unite, through resource mobilisation and campaigning with the policy makers to push through the Doctor's vision. The Sevatidevi App is a healthcare solution that works even with 2G data, and that, by itself, is revolutionary.

In my assessment, the Doctor has put in all the hard-work towards a great service to the nation. The implementation of the Project will enable our country to lead the change that can overcome all pitfalls and handicaps that have, for so long, rendered the pursuit of universal healthcare an impossible dream.

The Doctor a man on a mission. And I feel truly privileged that I could join hands with him in his futuristic vision.

Welcome to the Future!"

Dr. Naresh Gupta
MBBS, DOMS, FCLI
Eyes Specialist, General Physician and Surgeon
UNI Health Centre, Lovely Professional University, Jalandhar, India

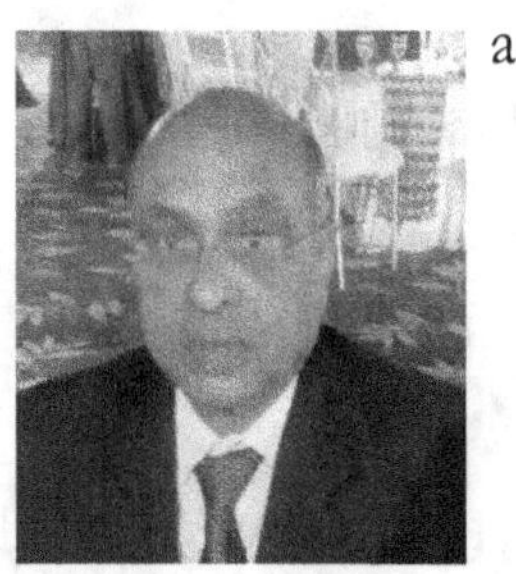

" Arvind was my shy but serious classmate at M G M C o l l e g e, Jamshedpur.

In my humble and honest opinion, his idea of T e l e - M e d i c i n e is revolutionary. And over the years that I've seen the Project blueprint evolve, I've come to believe that most diseases can be cured through Arvind's concept of *Healthcare at Home* for the poor.

Given that it really f a c i l i t a t e s q u i c k communication between patients and doctors/ healthcare professionals, Tele-Medicine is the need of the hour.

I believe that the implementation of this futuristic project through a strong IT network will play yeoman role in advancing the science and reach of Medicine. Satellite DMCs must be set up in the maximum geographies to cover all bases. The Doctor(s) posted at the Digital Medical Centres that are state-of-art self sustained diagnostic units, equipped with X-ray, Ultrasound and other lab equipments will help to accurately diagnose and instantly act on the test results.

Seeing the benefits for the rural people of having 'Specialists' available at the doorstep; other states, not to mention other nations, will automatically take it up like a good practice. Of course, implementation of this project will require a lot of effort. But Arvind has dared to tread the

unbeaten path. It's truly a
wonderful mission.

Arvind's Project
has to be implemented
without loss of time. And

out of dedication. "

Mr. Pradeep Ganatra
Ex Medical Director,
Bidada Sarvodaya Trust
Hospital, Bidada, Tal
Mandvi, Kutch, Gujarat &
Ex Coordinator,
Jayaramdas Patel Academic
Centre Muljibhai Patel
Urological Hospital,
Nadiad, Gujarat, India

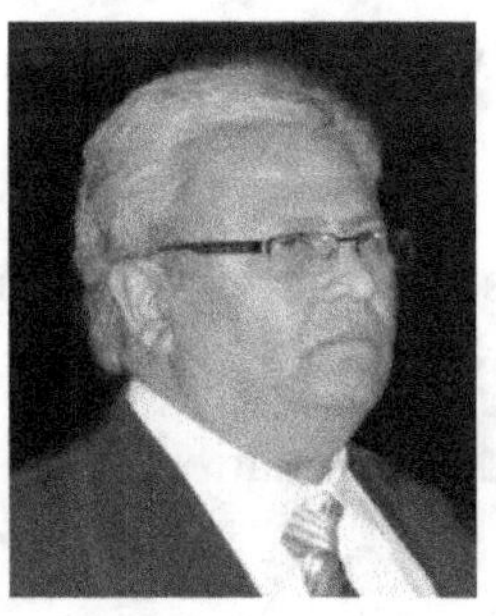

"   Arvind and I graduated from the Medical College, Jamshedpur the same year and we've continued to be friends ever since.

The subject of Tele-Medicine has always been especially close to my heart as I've been variously involved in the formulation of various public policies and guidelines released by the government on the matter. The Indian government came up with guidelines, video and audio message titled 'Tele Medicine Practice Guidelines', back in 2002; but the onset of Covid revealed that while the technology was there, it lacked appropriate harnessing. Hence, renewed effort ensued and the government released a revamped 'Tele Medicine Practice Guidelines' on 25th March 2020 at the Indian Medical Council.

From the wake of the new millennium, the situation on the ground has changed quite a lot now. And given the present state of world affairs, *Affordability* has emerged as an increasingly important question.

Arvind's Project is genuinely viable and technologically sound. But we need to move fast on this. It offers a unified mode of healthcare delivery to millions and millions of people across the country who are struggling to afford quality healthcare.

Once we get started, I can see more support pouring in. Also different and subsidiary professions may find their spaces to join in under Arvind's model. Suddenly, this will effect a big change and be quite a Revolution. But mind, that this will also bring about a massive change in the status quo, as do all big ideas. So, some convincing (campaign-building towards mobilising opinion) may be necessary to get the State to get behind the Idea. Also, companies and non-governmental organisations will play a very important role in pushing forward the idea and driving social change! Liaison officers who are politically active may prove especially useful here.

Once the ball starts rolling, results are quick and relief is immediate. It's about time we got started."

Dr. Rajesh Loomba
MBBS, MS, (ENT)
ENT Specialist, Ambala,
India

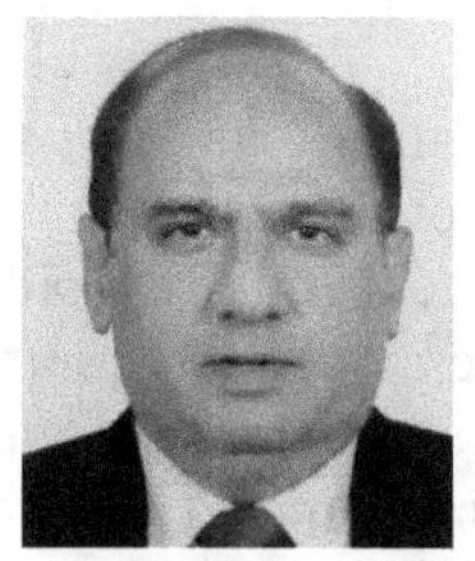

"   I first met Arvind at SD College, Ambala. Then we were together at MGM Medical College, Jamshedpur and our friendship really bloomed. We used to hang out together quite a lot!

It's a grand thing that Arvind is doing - Delivering Health to the poorest of the poor.

Arvind has been at it since 1968. He was way ahead of his time. I remember how he would hold the audience captive through his ideas and vision when he took the stage to make presentations. Am especially reminded of the huge response to his presentation and live demo at the Chandigarh CII Conference that was chaired by Shri J P Nadda (the then health Minister of Himachal Pradesh) and attended by the governments of Punjab, Haryana and Chandigarh, amongst others.

Through a video presentation, Arvind demonstrated Remote Robotic surgery, showing demo of a 360 degree MRI. He was assisted by his colleagues from Rikshospitalet, Norway and from the US where the live patient examination of eyes, ears, nose, throat and skin was conducted real time! Arvind wielded his stethoscope to examine the patient's heart even though they were oceans apart.

He demonstrated before the doctors, experts and government. And he did this almost 40 years back, when the Internet was just about beginning to come in. The conference was a great success.

A half decade ago, Arvind was making electric blankets. He is a very strong innovator. And always far ahead of the time.

I have had the privilege of following his journey closely and I feel, it's about time the government begins to promote the Project. Wake up and take up the Project on war footing, facilitate its execution through every possible technology including drones (especially useful after the lessons Covid-19 taught us).

We need to build some serious seed funding that can actively steer the course of the Project and create a holistic setup for procuring and delivering healthcare 'Amazon' style. Arvind has been on the job these last 4 decades.

And he's a genius, quite an Einstein of the time."

Dr. Rakesh Sahni
MD.FACC.FSCAI
Cardiologist and
Interventional cardiologist
Sahani Heart Centre
53-59, Westfield Ave, Clark
MJ 07066United States

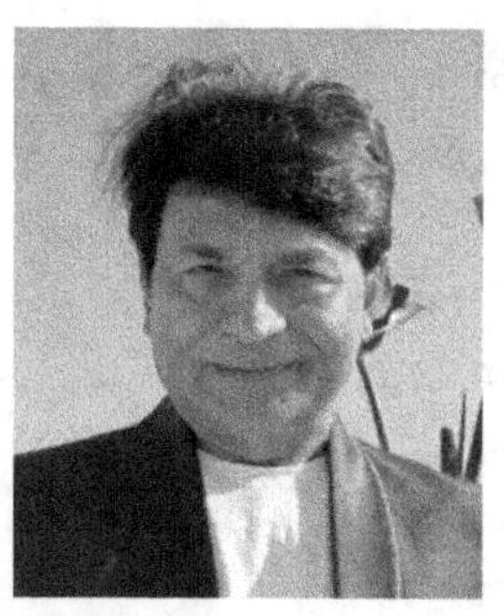

" Our story begins by sharing the same hostel room in MGM Medical College, Jamshedpur. And over the years, we've continued to remain in close touch across the oceans! Arvind was always very innovative and extraordinarily intelligent. Amongst his many virtues are discipline, determination and hard work. I've learnt much from him, including his tenacity for sticking it out despite the odds.

Albeit rudimentarily, 1950s saw the start of Tele-Medicine in Massachusetts, US. In the remotest places that could not make it to the big cities.

Arvind is perhaps one of the firsts who identified that a large population size, illiteracy and lack of communication are major challenges thwarting healthcare delivery for us in India and indeed, anywhere in the world. Through his model, Arvind has revolutionised Healthcare. Making Super-Specialist consultation available to so many people in remote places or without the means to access healthcare. He's perhaps, for the first and only time, worked out the infrastructure in terms of an elaborate layout that provides for a remote but instant system of Healthcare. This is what can be termed the 'Great Revolution in Healthcare'.

What Arvind's Tele-Medicine project will do is give us a 3 am emergency system that continues to work in normal times.

Misinformation is rampant in India. And we need to guard against it. Tele-Medicine is a very practical solution. Healthcare is a multi-billion dollar industry and over the last four decades, we've only experienced a growth boom. As we go into the future, Healthcare especially, is going to proliferate. Somebody has to go out there and implement it in the best possible way for India. In my conversations with Arvind across our distinct time zones and political worlds, I've found him relentlessly working on this unique aspect. His passion for the Project is infectious. Naturally, with all the groundwork that he's done over the years and his passionate zeal, Arvind's been a true crusader of Tele-Medicine through the years. Having kickstarted this mission for India, he's the ideal person to spearhead it for the rest of the world.

It's a win-win situation for everyone. The state of technology is now finally ready to host a continuum of care. Covid or no Covid. Rain or Shine. Tele-Medicine will establish a true continuum of care. It will remove the barriers of time, distance and money. Tele-Medicine is here to stay. We need to join in the conversation to make this into a movement.

All strength to Arvind!"

Thy right is to work only, but never to its
fruits; let not the fruit-of-action be thy
motive, nor let thy attachment be to
inaction.

Bhagavad Gita, 2:47

About the Author

Dr. Arvind Aggarwal   is a widely-respected Doctor,
 committed   towards ensuring accessible, affordable and
quality Healthcare to the last person in the last village
of the world

His concept of remote healthcare with its detailed plan
of public outreach has created ripples with very many
state governments in India as well as global leaders. His
vision stands out in its reach beyond the immediate crisis
to focus on long t erm growth   and stability, offering a
comprehensive blueprint for a truly Digital Healthcare
system emanating from India, for the World, in the 21st
century.